Sex, Drugs and Young People

All over the world, young people have been the focus of moral panic concerning sex and sexuality, illicit drug and substance use. While there is global concern about teenage pregnancy and rising rates of sexually transmitted infection and HIV/AIDS, a not uncommon view is that young people are irresponsible pleasure-seekers who live only for the present.

Sex, Drugs and Young People calls into question the mainstream assumptions about adolescence and youth that underlie many of our understandings of teenagers and young adults. The book provides a view of the transition to adulthood as not merely biologically and developmentally driven, but rather as socially and culturally shaped.

Bringing together a range of cross-national contributions, the book examines similarities and differences that mark both sexuality and drug use among young people in different social and cultural settings. In doing so, it allows the reader to build a clearer understanding of the challenges that must be faced in fields such as public health and education if we are to develop programmes that really serve the needs of young people.

Sex, Drugs and Young People will be of interest to professionals working with young people and is suitable for a wide range of multidisciplinary courses covering areas such as human sexuality, sex education, public health, education and social work.

Peter Aggleton is Professor in Education and Director of the Thomas Coram Research Unit at the Institute of Education, University of London.

Andrew Ball is Senior Strategy and Operations Advisor in the World Health Organization's Department of HIV/AIDS, Geneva.

Purnima Mane is Director of the Department of Policy, Evidence and Partnerships in the Joint United Nations Programme on HIV/AIDS (UNAIDS), Geneva.

Sexuality, Culture and Health series

Edited by

Peter Aggleton, Institute of Education, University of London, UK
Richard Parker, Columbia University, New York, USA
Sonia Correa, ABIA, Rio de Janeiro, Brazil
Gary Dowsett, La Trobe University, Melbourne, Australia
Shirley Lindenbaum, City University of New York, USA

This new series of books offers cutting-edge analysis, current theoretical perspectives and up-to-the minute ideas concerning the interface between sexuality, public health, human rights, culture and social development. It adopts a global and interdisciplinary perspective in which the needs of poorer countries are given equal status to those of richer nations. The books are written with a broad range of readers in mind, and will be invaluable to students, academics and those working in policy and practice. The series aims to serve as a spur to practical action in an increasingly globalised world.

Sex, Drugs and Young People

International perspectives

Edited by
Peter Aggleton, Andrew Ball
and Purnima Mane

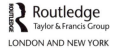

LONDON AND NEW YORK

First published 2006
by Routledge
2 Park Square, Milton Park, Abingdon, Oxon, OX14 4RN

Simultaneously published in the USA and Canada
by Routledge
270 Madison Avenue, New York, NY 10016

Routledge is an imprint of the Taylor & Francis Group

© 2006 Peter Aggleton, Andrew Ball and Purnima Mane

Typeset in Sabon by
Keystroke, Jacaranda Lodge, Wolverhampton
Printed and bound in Great Britain by
TJ International Ltd, Padstow, Cornwall

British Library Cataloguing in Publication Data
A catalogue record for this book is available from the British Library

Library of Congress Cataloging in Publication Data
Sex, drugs and young people : international perspectives / edited by Peter Aggleton,
Andrew Ball and Purnima Mane.
     p. cm.
  Includes bibliographical references and index.
  ISBN 0-415-32877-2 (hardback : alk. paper) – ISBN 0-415-32878-0 (pbk. : alk. paper)
 1. Youth–Sexual behavior–Cross-cultural studies. 2. Youth–Drug use–Cross-cultural
studies. I. Aggleton, Peter. II. Ball, Andrew. III. Mane, Purnima N.
  HV5824.Y68S47 2005
  306.7'0835–dc22   2005015912

ISBN10: 0–415–32877–2   ISBN13: 9–78–0–415–32877–7 (hbk)
ISBN10: 0–415–32878–0   ISBN13: 9–78–0–415–32878–4 (pbk)

Disclaimer

The findings, interpretations and views expressed in this book are entirely those of the
author(s) and do not necessarily reflect official policy or positions of the Joint United
Nations Programme on HIV/AIDS (UNAIDS) or the World Health Organization (WHO).

For Kim Rivers

Contents

Contributors

Peter Aggleton is Director of the Thomas Coram Research Unit at the Institute of Education, University of London. The author and editor of over twenty books in the field of health promotion, he has acted as a senior adviser and consultant to UNAIDS, UNESCO, UNICEF, WHO and a wide range of international agencies.

Anthony Arcuri is a doctoral student in counselling psychology at Macquarie University and a Research Officer at the Ted Noffs Foundation in Sydney.

Andrew Ball trained as a drug and alcohol physician and has worked in the areas of drug dependence treatment, HIV/AIDS and sexually transmitted infections, and adolescent health. He is Senior Strategy and Operations Advisor in the WHO Department of HIV/AIDS. Since joining WHO in 1991 he has supported work on young people, HIV/AIDS and substance use in a wide range of countries.

Sandra Bullock is an Assistant Professor in the Department of Health Studies and Gerontology at the University of Waterloo, Canada. Her research focuses on the patterns and social consequences of alcohol and drug use among young adults, with a primary focus on the relationship between substance use and participation in unsafe sex.

Chris Castle is Senior Programme Specialist for HIV/AIDS and Education with UNESCO in Paris. Prior to taking up his present post, he worked with HealthLink Worldwide, the Horizons Program and the International HIV/AIDS Alliance.

Jan Copeland is a Senior Lecturer at the National Drug and Alcohol Research Centre at the University of New South Wales. She has conducted research into a range of alcohol and other drug-related issues over the past sixteen years including treatment for women, juvenile justice and treatment outcome evaluation.

Linda Eriksson is Programme Officer for HIV and Gender at the International Organization for Migration in Colombia. She has worked on development, emergency response and HIV and mobility issues in Latin America for the past eight years.

Martin Foreman is an independent consultant working in Bangkok. He is the author of many studies on the social causes and consequences of the global HIV/AIDS epidemic.

Dennis Gray is an Associate Professor and Deputy Director of the National Drug Research Institute at Curtin University of Technology in Perth, Western Australia. He has a background in medical anthropology and public health and has published widely on indigenous health and substance use issues.

Danielle Grondin is Director of the Migration Health Department at the International Organization for Migration. She is responsible for the development and planning of health policy and strategy to promote migration health. Prior to taking up her present post, she worked for the Canadian Department of Citizenship and Immigration.

Mary Haour-Knipe is Senior Adviser on Migration and HIV/AIDS at the International Organization for Migration, where she provides technical support and guidance for development of IOM's HIV/AIDS-related programmes worldwide. She is the author or editor of numerous publications in the fields of migration and HIV/AIDS, migration and families, and social equity and health.

John Howard has worked in education, juvenile justice, adolescent psychiatry and university settings. He is currently Director of Clinical Services, Training and Research for the Ted Noffs Foundation in Sydney, which works with young people experiencing significant difficulties associated with substance use.

Neil Hunt is Director of Research for KCA, a Senior Research Associate at the European Institute of Social Services at the University of Kent, and an honorary Research Fellow at the Centre for Research on Drugs and Health Behaviour, Imperial College London.

Carol Jenkins is a medical anthropologist, currently working as an independent consultant on AIDS and related issues. She previously worked with the United States Agency for International Development, the US National Institutes of Health, Family Health International, CARE Bangladesh, and the Papua New Guinea Institute of Medical Research.

Deborah Keys is a research fellow at the Key Centre for Women's Health in Society at the University of Melbourne, Australia. She is a sociologist whose research interests encompass identity and the self, sexuality, youth, drugs, and sexual health. She is currently engaged in research with young people experiencing homelessness.

Purnima Mane is Director of the Department of Policy, Evidence and Partnerships in the Joint United Nations Programme on AIDS (UNAIDS), Geneva, Switzerland. Over the last twenty-five years, she has worked on reproductive and sexual health, gender issues, and AIDS in academic institutions and international organizations in India, the United States of America and Switzerland.

Rita M. Melendez is an Assistant Professor in the Human Sexuality Studies Program and a Research Associate at the Center for Research on Gender and Sexuality at San Francisco State University. She researches how gender dynamics contribute to HIV risk behaviours.

Cheryl Overs was founder and coordinator of the Prostitutes Collective of Victoria and the Scarlet Alliance, Australia's national federation of sex worker organizations. She currently works at the International HIV/AIDS Alliance providing technical support to focused HIV prevention programmes.

Marian Pitts is Director of the Australian Research Centre in Sex, Health and Society at LaTrobe University, Melbourne. She is part of the research team that conducts a nationwide survey of Australian secondary school students. This survey, conducted every five years, tracks changes in young people's sexual activity and examines patterns of drinking and drug use.

Kim Rivers has until recently worked as a Research Officer within the Thomas Coram Research Unit at the Institute of Education, University of London. Her interests include young people and sexual health, masculinities and HIV-related vulnerability, and the evaluation of innovative health programmes. She has extensive international field experience in Eastern Europe and Asia.

Robin Room is a Professor and Director at the Centre for Social Research on Alcohol and Drugs at Stockholm University. He has studied patterns and problems in general populations, the social ecology of treatment, and cultural and policy changes and their effects, particularly for alcohol but also for drugs and gambling.

Doreen Rosenthal is Director of the Key Centre for Women's Health in Society at the University of Melbourne, Australia. Her research interests include adolescent sexuality and sexual health, gender and the social construction of sexuality and adolescent homelessness.

Sherry Saggers is Foundation Professor of Applied Social Research and Director of the Centre for Social Research at Edith Cowan University in Western Australia. She has published widely on indigenous health and substance misuse issues, including a comparative study of indigenous substance use in Australia, Canada and New Zealand.

Phillipa Strempel was, at the time of writing, a Research Associate at the National Drug Research Institute, Curtin University of Technology. She was also a co-author of the report *Indigenous Drug and Alcohol Projects: Elements of Best Practice* published by the Australian National Council on Drugs.

Deborah L. Tolman is Director of the Center for Research on Gender and Sexuality (CRGS) and Professor of Human Sexuality Studies at San Francisco State University. A developmental psychologist, she studies constructions of gender and experiences of sexuality among adolescent girls and boys in the USA.

Acknowledgements

The editors would like to express their appreciation to Geeta Rao Gupta for her helpful comments on elements of the text, and to Fiona Thirlwell for her editorial assistance and support.

Chapter 1

Introduction

Peter Aggleton, Andrew Ball and Purnima Mane

Put together the words 'sex' and 'young people' and there are the makings of controversy. Add the word 'drugs', and there is a specially potent mix. In combination, the three terms – sex, drugs and adolescence – have laid the foundations for early twenty-first century understandings of young people, their circumstances and needs. On the television and in the news, it is not uncommon to hear the claim that young people are risk-takers who live only for the moment. In more academic literature and in government reports, young people are portrayed as sexually irresponsible and prone to alcohol and substance abuse. In the eyes of pundits, young people are said to be ego-centric, unable to adjust to the wider demands of the family and community. As a result of this, doctors, health and social care professionals, families and friends face the difficult task of shepherding wayward individuals back to the safe and narrow.

But where did such ideas about young people come from and do they offer a reasonable portrayal of young people's lives and needs? G. Stanley Hall, one of the founders of developmental psychology, was one of the first to write about such ideas in his book *Adolescence: Its Psychology and its Relations to Physiology, Anthropology, Sociology, Sex, Crime, Religion, and Education* (Hall 1904). This two volume 1,300 page tome, not only established 'adolescence' as a unique stage of development, but also imbued this period of life with negative and problematic characteristics. Hall's somewhat deprecatory ideas were later taken up in the work of psycho-analytic writers such as Erik Erikson (1968/1974) who saw adolescence as a period of crisis resolving the tension between identity formation and 'identity confusion'. For numerous writers thereafter, a key developmental task associated with adolescence was that of integration into the community. Without such integration there can only be maladjustment, disturbance and difficulty. Such are the historical foundations upon which numerous modern day understandings of young people have been built.

But do such images offer a realistic portrayal of young people and their needs? The assumption that adolescence is a universal stage of turmoil and confusion to be passed through en route to a more balanced adulthood has been deeply questioned by the work of anthropologists such as Margaret Mead (1928/1961). Her book entitled *Coming of Age in Samoa* questioned the inevitability of the 'storm and stress' (see Hechinger and Hechinger 1963) normally equated with adolescence. For Mead, the problems and conflicts associated with youth as a stage of life were as much a consequence of the economic and social organization of society in general, as the individual. In non-Western societies such as Samoa, youth and early adulthood were characterized by harmony and balance. In other societies such as the USA and Europe, they were associated with problems. For Mead and her followers the 'problems of adolescence' are cultural constructions with roots in history, the economy and the societal arrangements that deny young people opportunities and refuse to take their perspectives and experiences seriously.

In recent years, writers such as Manning (1983), Offer and Schonert-Reichl (1992), and Maira and Soep (2004) have pointed to some of the myths about adolescence that require critical scrutiny. These include the notion that normal adolescent development is tumultuous, when for many young people it is not. An over-reliance on evidence from clinical samples of severely disturbed young people led psychologists of the 1950s and 1960s (e.g. Freud 1958; Blos 1962) to conclude that *all* young people were disturbed.

Likewise, the idea that adolescence is a time of increased emotionality and frequent mood change is now questioned, with recent research showing that adolescents are on average no more moody than those who are younger (Larson and Lampman-Petraitis 1989). The notion that puberty is universally experienced as a negative event by young people has similarly been shown to be false (Brooks-Gunn and Reiter 1990), as has the belief that adolescent thought is immature and childlike (Keating 1990).

While negative images and attitudes towards young people persist, paralleling dominant discourses of sickness, deviance and difficulty are those of a quite different kind. In the writings of early twentieth century reformers such Jane Addams, for example, it is possible to find an altogether more sympathetic appreciation of young people. Where her other contemporaries saw difficulties and problems, Addams saw confidence and hope – the ability to stand free from fear, and the capacity to 'create order out of casualty, beauty out of confusion, and justice, kindliness and mercy out of cruelty and inconsiderate pressure' (Addams 1909). Such views have their parallel in the programmes and actions of modern day youth movements all over the world as well as internationally agreed upon human rights instruments such as the UN Convention on the Rights of the Child.

These contrasting views of young people and their needs, the first pathological and vilificatory, the second more understanding of young people's circumstances and needs, constitute the poles around which adults have been encouraged to understand the actions and behaviours of young people all over the world. Yet to our mind both perspectives run the risk of misreading the situation. Neither, for example, takes cognizance of the fact that not all young people are the same – the risks and opportunities facing individuals vary in relation to social background, gender, sexuality, culture and ethnicity among other factors (see, for example, Epstein 1998; Skelton and Valentine 1998). Neither approach has much to say either about the broader cultural and social context in which young people live their lives. Nor do such frameworks integrate the light and shade in young people's lives by recognizing, for example, that the same young person may be vigorous, positive, constructive and forward looking at one moment in time, but negative, withdrawn and at risk, the next.

In responding to these concerns, and in offering the foundations for a new and more positive international health agenda, this book seeks to offer a more realistic portrayal of young people, their circumstances, experiences and needs – especially in relation to sex and drugs. Its starting point lies in recognition that young people are, above all, a *heterogeneous group*. They differ from one another in terms of social background, ambition, interests, opportunities and faith – sometimes in small ways and sometimes very considerably. Only rarely is their social behaviour – like that of adults – over-determined by their biology. More usually, their actions are influenced by political and legal factors, social meanings and motivations, and the economic opportunities available to them. Young people are however more than 'individuals' in the free-floating sense of being cut off and separated from society. Instead, their experiences and opportunities are deeply *structured* by gender, ethnicity/race, class, age and sexuality among other factors. In almost every country of the world, the circumstances and needs of young women differ systematically from those of young men; issues of age and class are important in making sense of young people's experiences and responses; and sexuality, economic status, disability and other factors open up, and restrict, opportunities for health.

It is crucial to recognize also that young people are the *bearers of rights*. The rights enshrined in the UN Convention on the Rights of the Child and allied declarations should in our view be the starting point for policy and programme development. But taking these international commitments seriously carries with it major responsibilities for adults. It involves taking seriously what young people say and do, it involves providing opportunities for young people to express their views on matters relevant to their own lives, it involves listening carefully, and it involves taking young people's per--spectives into account when planning and providing services. Doing this encourages the adoption of what might be described as a *positive approach* to understanding young people and health, and to responding to their potential. Such a perspective is in contrast to the dominant paradigm, which persists in seeing young people as 'collections of difficulties and problems' that require treatment, supervision and intervention. This new more positive approach also calls for partnership and participation. As the contributions in this volume show, the promotion of young people's health is best facilitated by a supportive and inclusive response. Too often in the past, programmes have failed because they have sought to blame young people rather than listen to them. In parallel, they have offered opportunities for tokenistic rather than genuine participation.

Via a series of linked chapters, and with a global focus, our goal is to explore the implications of the above premises for two key aspects of young people's lives – their sexual and reproductive health and their engagement with both licit and illicit substance use. These chapters also aim to examine the inter-relationships between these two phenomena. We begin with a focus on what might be described as the structuring of vulnerability – or the manner in which young people *systematically* find it difficult to maximize their sexual and reproductive health and to cope in societies where drugs are prevalent.

Globally, the opportunities and choices available to young people are severely restricted by human poverty and by its intersections with gender. Lack of access to economic resources and the power that comes with these, is associated with a wide range of sexual health problems – especially for young women. These include early childbearing and sexually transmitted infections including HIV. For poverty, rural to urban migration and home-lessness are also associated with substance use and involvement in sex work. In chapter 2, **Kim Rivers, Peter Aggleton** and **Andrew Ball** discuss these factors, exploring the interface between poverty, gender and education, among other factors, and their implications for substance use, and for sexual and mental health.

Issues of gender are taken up in more detail in chapter 3. Here, **Rita M. Melendez** and **Deborah L. Tolman** move beyond the individual to consider the patterned nature of young women's social disadvantage and its implications for sexual health. Drawing on case study material from the USA and from Nepal, as well as on the academic and programmatic literature, they point to the systematically structured nature of this disadvantage to advance the notion of vulnerability in making sense of young people's experiences. Their work points once more to the intersections between gender and poverty as determinants of the opportunities available to young people and the risks, including gender and sexual violence, that both women and men may face. They use case studies from Nigeria, the UK and the USA to point to heightened vulnerability for many young women and demonstrate how programmatic advances can be made to respond to diverse groups of young people's rights and needs.

Chapter 4, by **Carol Jenkins**, examines issues of race, culture and ethnicity in relation to young people's use of licit and illicit drugs, as well as the links between sex and substance use. The use of mind-altering drugs has an ancient history. Societies all over the world have found that certain plants or other substances affect the mind in ways that are valued for their capacity to transform perceptions, moods or emotions. For the majority of young people, trying out different psychoactive substances is more of a social activity than anything else and may not be associated with low self-esteem, deviance or criminality. A better understanding is required both of normative patterns of substance use, the 'functionality' or otherwise of specific forms of use, and the factors associated with serious harm, both for the self and for others. Harm reduction for drug users has shown clear success in reducing health and social risks. But in many parts of the world, governments wish to enforce a 'no drugs–no sex' policy for young people. Yet, there is little in human history to suggest these are reasonable or attainable goals, and by denying young people access to the full range of options, such policies are in fact detrimental in terms of protecting young people from drug-related problems or sexually transmitted infections.

The second part of this book looks more specifically at young people's sexual and substance use practices, as well as the relationships between them. In chapter 5, **Deborah Keys, Doreen Rosenthal** and **Marian Pitts** examine the links between sexual behaviour, sexual well-being and sexual vulnerability within a framework that stresses the positive potential of young people as sexual beings. They examine variations and trends in age of first sexual intercourse and the push and pull factors involved. Young people embark on sexual careers for many reasons, ranging from the affective to the financial. Cultural and gender factors exert significant influences on meaning, with young men being often more likely to cite pleasure, desire and physical satisfaction and women, love, intimacy or desire for a close relationship. The authors conclude that early sexual initiation is not necessarily a problem in itself. Rather, lack of information, education and/or support may lead to unwelcome outcomes for those who experience an early sexual debut. A broader definition of sex is called for in making sense of young people's experiences, which recognizes the importance of masturbation and same-sex practices, as well as the potential of sex to be a pleasurable and positive aspect of a young person's life.

In chapter 6, **Neil Hunt** shifts the focus slightly to look at patterns of substance use. All over the world, concern has been expressed about young people's use of illicit drugs such as cannabis, inhalants, sedatives, amphetamine-type stimulants, cocaine and heroin. Social surveys consistently identify drug use as a widespread activity among young people. Usually, it occurs within a variably-sized minority of the population. However, studies of young offenders, children excluded from school, children in care or regular club-goers commonly find that drug use is, statistically, the norm rather than the exception. In this kind of situation, what should be our response? First, we need to understand the diversity of phenomena involved – and the range of factors that may lead to involvement in substance use. Second, there is a need for 'intelligent intervention', as Hunt describes it, programmes and actions provided in contexts and with a focus that responds to young people's diverse circumstances and needs.

Chapter 7, by **John Howard** and **Anthony Arcuri**, builds upon such concern by examining the situation of drug use among same-sex attracted young people. The chapter emphasizes the 'meaningfulness' of different forms of substance use, and the need for focused programmes of different kinds. It also highlights the special circumstances of same-sex attracted young people, the discrimination that many experience, and the capacity of drugs to temporarily alleviate the pain of this abuse. While most same-sex attracted young people survive their teenage years minimally scarred and resilient, a minority do not, and some may find that substance use enhances vulnerability to sex-related risks. Exposure to a range of role models may decrease isolation by providing examples of resilience and coping, and both specialist and non-specialist youth services have an important role in educating individuals and promoting health.

In chapter 8, the focus shifts to patterns of alcohol use. **Sandra Bullock** and **Robin Room** examine three broad questions: what is known about patterns of alcohol consumption among young people around the world; how has the consumption of alcohol by young people been conceptualized in the literature; and how does drinking relate to other activities such as violence and sex? Their chapter reveals something of the diversity in drinking behaviour among young people internationally, as well as its relationship to societal norms, interpersonal relationships and societal level structural forces including regulation and the law. They find evidence however of an increasing similarity in young people's drinking patterns across countries, linked to the rise of club and other recreational cultures. Yet alcohol-related changes in social behaviour vary considerably across countries and settings, making it foolish to link alcohol consumption unproblematically with violence and/or sexual risk-taking. Their chapter ends with a discussion of programmatic implications including fiscal measures as well as efforts to bring about change in culturally based attitudes and expectations.

The third and final part of this book focuses on the special circumstances in which some young people may find themselves. In chapter 9, **Cheryl Overs** and **Chris Castle** examine the interface between drug and sexual health risks, including HIV. They stress that the links between substance use, sex work and vulnerability for young people are not simple or amenable to generalization. The drugs themselves, the context in which they are used and the way in which sex is exchanged for money or other resources, all influence risk and vulnerability to HIV. To develop effective policy and strategies, we need to look at a broad range of sexual and drug-taking behaviours across a range of contexts. This requires us to understand the diversity of reasons why young people may sell or trade sex, and why they become involved in drug use. It also requires respect for young people themselves and the essential contribution they can make to addressing the vulnerabilities they face. National authorities and service providers must find ways of overcoming overly compartmentalized and stigmatizing programmes, as well as those that fail to deliver comprehensive and easily accessed services in which the service user is firmly at the centre.

Chapter 10, by **Mary Haour-Knipe, Linda Eriksson** and **Danielle Grondin,** considers the special circumstances of young migrants and refugees. It describes the reasons why young people migrate and the contexts of vulnerability present in the country of origin, in transit and at the point of destination. Norms and behaviours may shift when a young person is transposed from one place to another, and although many young people navigate such journeys very well, some may find themselves vulnerable to exploitation by employers and by those who deal in the trafficking of drugs and of human beings. Young migrants and refugees have many of the same needs for health and other services as other young people, including health promotion and help for drug-related problems. But access to services is often difficult, and hindrances can include language barriers, lack of information and of trust, and services that are culturally inappropriate. Successful responses include the development and provision of services that are both youth-friendly and migrant-friendly. They include measures to ensure access to housing, schools, health and social services regardless of legal status; and to improve conditions so that people do not have to relocate against their will in the first place, or can do so with as much protection as possible.

Over 20 million people serve in the armed forces across the world, and each year over a million young people enter or leave military service. The world's armed forces share many similarities – in addition to being relatively young and overwhelmingly male, they are hierarchical and highly mobile. There is evidence that military life can have a significant impact on young people's social, psychological and sexual development; that in many, if not most, military forces young people are more sexually active than civilians of the same age; that a significant proportion of young soldiers drink heavily; and that, with some exceptions, illicit drug use is probably not widespread among young soldiers. Chapter 11, by **Martin Foreman,** explores some of these issues and their consequences for young people's sexual and mental health. He concludes that while some young people are well suited to military life and benefit from it; others are physically or mentally scarred. Whatever the basis under which they serve, young people in many militaries fail to develop healthy attitudes and behaviour towards sex, alcohol and recreational drugs. Education and support need to be developed and expanded within this context.

Globally, more than a million young people have been deprived of their liberty by law enforcement authorities and officials. Settings in which they may be detained include adult jails, juvenile detention centres, community group homes, re-education camps, labour camps, refugee camps, orphanages, and mandatory residential mental health or drug treatment programmes. What kinds of risks do young people face in such situations and what steps can be taken to protect their rights? In chapter 12,

Jan Copeland, John Howard and Anthony Arcuri examine these concerns. They document high levels of violence in detention, the systematic failure to guarantee legal representation and fair hearing, physical and sexual abuse and substance use. Detained young people may have elevated exposure to drug, sex and tattoo/body piercing risk factors for diseases such as HIV and hepatitis C, yet few efforts are currently made at harm reduction or diversion away from custodial environments. The need for developmentally appropriate forms of service delivery that address the structural determinants of substance use and sexual vulnerability both before and after detention, alongside efforts to promote the prosocial development and integration of young offenders, is stressed.

In the final chapter in this volume, Sherry Saggers, Dennis Gray, and Phillipa Strempel focus on indigenous young people. While heterogeneous and geographically widespread, indigenous people share a common history of colonialism, dispossession and exclusion. Recent research has also shown that despite their diversity, indigenous young people are more likely to be sexually active and at an earlier age than their non-indigenous counterparts. Use of contraception is likely to be lower, birth complications higher, and rates of sexually transmitted infections higher still. Despite the higher prevalence of drug problems among indigenous than in non-indigenous populations – the majority of indigenous people use drugs without problems. In reviewing programmatic options, the authors conclude that the best protection for indigenous young people is to be part of families and communities which have a strong stake in both their own cultures and future, as well as in mainstream society. In countries such as Australia, Canada, New Zealand and the USA much still needs to be done to symbolically and materially address the injustices of the colonial past, in order to provide indigenous young people with the foundations for health and well-being.

Regardless of their context or focus, several themes recur throughout this book. They include concern for the diversity of young people, their circumstances and needs; the structured vulnerability to ill health that many face on grounds of social background, gender, sexuality, ethnicity and race; the value of listening carefully to what young people say and including them fully in the development of programmes; and the importance of adopting a rights-based approach in meeting young people's sexual and drug-related health needs. Too often in the past, young people have been stereotyped and vilified – often under the guise of doing what is best for them. Now is the time for a fresh approach: not one that romanticizes the power of youth, but one that recognizes the inherent dignity of *every* human being and their right to proper participation in health.

With these messages in mind, we hope that readers will themselves feel empowered to learn from young people and to sometimes be surprised. For too long, half-truths, taboos and distortions have gone unchallenged when it comes to young people, sex and drugs. In consequence, policies have been ill thought out and programmes have suffered. Now is the time to begin to put things right. We hope you feel inspired by what you read, and encouraged by the many opportunities that exist to develop more positive appreciations of young people, their circumstances and needs.

Peter Aggleton   March 2005
London

Andrew Ball
Geneva

Purnima Mane
Geneva

References

Addams, J. (1909) *The Spirit of Youth and the City Streets*. New York, Macmillan.

Blos, P. (1962) *On Adolescence*. New York, Free Press.

Brooks-Gunn, J. and Reiter, E. (1990) The role of pubertal processes in the early adolescent transition. In S. Feldman and G. Elliott (eds) *At the Threshold: The Developing Adolescent*. Cambridge, MA, Harvard University Press.

Epstein, J. (1998) *Youth Culture: Identity in a Postmodern World*. Oxford, Blackwell.

Erikson, E. (1968/1974) *Identity, Youth and Crisis*. New York, W.W. Norton.

Freud, A. (1958) Adolescence. *Psychoanalytic Study of the Child*, 13, 255–78.

Hall, G.S. (1904) *Adolescence: Its Psychology and its Relations to Physiology, Anthropology, Sociology, Sex, Crime, Religion and Education*. New York: Appleton Century Crofts.

Hechinger, F. and Hechinger, G. (1963) *Teenage Tyranny*. New York, William Morrow.

Keating, D. (1990) Adolescent thinking. In S. Feldman and G. Elliott (eds) *At the Threshold: The Developing Adolescent*. Cambridge, MA, Harvard University Press.

Larson, R. and Lampman-Petraitis, C. (1989) Daily emotional states as reported by children and adolescents. *Child Development*, 60, 1250–60.

Maira, S. and Soep, E. (2004) United States of Adolescence? Reconsidering US youth culture studies. *Young (Nordic Journal of Youth Research)*, 12, 245–69.

Manning, M. (1983) Three myths concerning adolescence. *Adolescence*, 18, 823–9.

Mead, M. (1928/1961) *Coming of Age in Samoa*. New York, William Morrow.

Offer, D. and Schonert-Reichl, K. (1992) Debunking the myths of adolescence: findings from recent research. *Journal of the American Academy of Child and Adolescent Psychiatry*, 31, 1003–14.

Skelton, T. and Valentine, G. (1998) *Cool Places: Geographies of Youth Cultures*. London, Routledge.

Part I

The structuring of vulnerability

Chapter 2

Young people, poverty and risk

Kim Rivers, Peter Aggleton and Andrew Ball

A review of the research and programmatic literature on young people, substance use and sexual health reveals a vast array of accounts and explanations of the risk factors young people face. These commonly include personal factors such as levels of knowledge; psychological factors, for example self-esteem and stress; family background, such as parental divorce and family violence; and cultural factors, including gender norms. However, relatively few studies deal directly or substantially with poverty and economic inequality. As a result, much research and many articles and papers concern themselves with the proximate causes of risk – lack of education, poor family cohesion, low self-esteem – without looking at the underlying causes of vulnerability including social inequality and poverty. In this chapter, the experiences of the world's poorest young people will be discussed in order to show how many of the widely agreed vulnerabilities for poor sexual and reproductive health, as well as some of those relating to drug use, are related to poverty.

Poverty, young people and risk

Overall, economic growth has led to a decrease in the numbers of people living in absolute poverty worldwide (Rao Gupta, Whelan and Allendorf 2003). However, in spite of this overall improvement, there is unevenness in the benefits of such growth: while some countries have reduced the numbers of people living in extreme poverty, in others poverty has been on the rise (UNFPA 2003). For example, up to a quarter of people in South Africa and Ethiopia, and up to a third in India are chronically poor – that is they have been poor over a long period, since birth or over generations (Chronic Poverty Research Centre 2002). Aside of this absolute poverty, qualitative approaches to poverty now take account of factors beyond income. The United Nations Development Programme measures deprivation in terms of basic human development as opposed to income poverty alone. Important factors to consider in this respect include having a short life, lack of basic education and lack of access to public and private resources

(UNDP 1997). Not surprisingly, one key area of human poverty relates to access to health.

The relationship between poverty and health is reasonably well understood:

> Poverty creates ill-health because it forces people to live in environments that make them sick . . . Poverty denies people access to reliable health services . . . creates illiteracy, leaving people poorly informed about health risks and forced into dangerous jobs.
>
> (WHO/WB 2002: 2)

As well as diseases related directly to nutrition and sanitation, and the infectious diseases that thrive in overcrowded environments, poor people do not enjoy optimum sexual and reproductive health – and in some parts of the world, they may also be more vulnerable to the risks associated with substance use. Rather than having a range of choices about sexual, reproductive and drug use behaviours, poor people routinely find themselves in situations that are injurious to their health: migrating from their families and usual conjugal partners to single-sex work environments; living on the streets where sex and drug use are means for survival and are used as coping strategies; selling or exchanging sex for food and shelter; and engaging in drug production and trafficking in the absence of any other means of survival. The patterning of the HIV epidemic over time bears this out. Research in southern Africa suggests that while in the early stages of the epidemic HIV transmission occurred at all economic and educational levels, in the later stages, people with greater access to money and education were more likely to change their behaviour as a result of HIV-prevention programmes, while those who were poorer remained vulnerable (Campbell 2003).

Young people in particular are vulnerable to both poverty and the sexual health and drug-related vulnerability it brings. Nearly half of all the people on earth are under the age of 25 and developing countries are home to 85 per cent of the world's young people (UNICEF, UNAIDS and WHO 2002). Half of these young people are poor, and one quarter – around 238 million – live on less than US$1 a day (UNFPA 2003). In many countries, poverty means that 'millions of young people are deprived of their most basic rights – the rights to shelter, health, education [and] care' (UNAIDS 2003: 6). It is widely agreed that young people generally have less access to information, skills, services and support than adults. However, poor young people, forced to live on the social and economic margins of society, have even less access to these resources than other young people. Not only are young people vulnerable to poverty, they 'also stand in the path of one of the deadliest epidemics ever' (UNAIDS 2003: 6). AIDS is known to be both a consequence and a cause of poverty. The influence of poverty in the spread of HIV is reflected in the differences in the epidemic affecting young people across different regions of the world. In sub-Saharan Africa, for example, more than eight and a half million young people aged between 15 and 24 years are estimated to be living with HIV, while in Western Europe, a much smaller number – around 90,000 young people – are believed to be infected (UNAIDS/WHO 2001).

While young people are not a homogeneous group, there are some commonalities in their experiences across different developing countries. Access to education is often limited, especially for girls, and levels of literacy are often low. Opportunities for employment may be restricted and decision-making is constrained by the necessity of meeting basic needs. Partly due to poverty, many young people are forced to endure situations – including discrimination, exploitation and social isolation – that render them vulnerable to unprotected sex, and drug and alcohol use (Burns et al. 2004). In some parts of the world, poor young people who are neither in school nor employed spend much of their time on the streets and within this context may find themselves vulnerable to drug use (Burns et al. 2004). There is a growing body of evidence that suggests that not just poverty, but stark economic inequalities have an impact on young people's sexual and drug-related behaviours. In some Eastern European countries, in particular, perhaps the majority of young people have found themselves suddenly propelled into relative poverty, while an élite minority have enjoyed material success. This has affected the way they feel about themselves and their future and consequently their sexual and substance-related behaviours.

Poor young people are often more vulnerable than adults to sexual and reproductive health threats and substance use. Adults across the world deny young people the information about sex and drugs that they need to protect their health (Aggleton and Rivers 1999), and age-related inequalities mean that young people do not have the same access to jobs as adults. Youth unemployment across the globe is twice as high as adult rates (Esim et al. 2001). As a result, young people often eke out a living on the margins – in the underground economy – through illicit trading, foraging for scrap items or even through involvement in criminal activities, including the drugs trade. Even when in legitimate employment, differentials in the wages paid to young people and adults mean that many young people find it hard to make ends meet. In a recent study, interviews with young garment factory workers in Cambodia revealed that employment did not provide them with enough to live on – they all worked overtime and were unable to take sick leave for fear of losing their job or wages (Maclean 1999).

Not surprisingly, young people living in poverty or facing the threat of poverty may be vulnerable to sexual exploitation through the need to trade or sell sex in order to survive (WHO 1998). Children and young people living in families surviving with the stresses and frustrations of poverty are also vulnerable to physical and sexual violence. In the recent World Health Organization report entitled *Dying for Change*, poor people interviewed across the world, including young people, revealed that children are widely subjected to abuse (WHO/WB 2002). Young people in Brazil, for example, described how their drunken fathers had beaten and raped them. Poor young people often have even less choice than poor adults: in many countries child labour, child trafficking, child prostitution and drug use among children and young people are a result of abuse, stress and precarious living arrangements.

Among the most vulnerable young people of all are those who face the triple jeopardy of being young, poor and female. Poor young women face even more limited economic opportunities than young men and are more likely to experience human poverty – that is limited access to resources such as education, information and health services – as well as having less control over decision-making. What is more, gender and youth intersect with ethnicity, caste and race to compound vulnerability. Ethnic, caste and racial minorities are disproportionately represented among the poor in every region of the world (Rao Gupta, Whelan and Allendorf 2003).

Poor young people's sexual and drug-related health

Almost one third of those living with HIV globally are under the age of 25. Of 4.2 million new adult infections in 2002, half were among young men and women (UNICEF, UNAIDS and WHO 2002). Young people aged 15–24 years have the highest incidence of sexually transmitted infections (STIs) of all age groups (Population Council 2002). Obstructed labour, HIV infection and chlamydia infection rank among the ten leading causes of disability-adjusted life years lost among young people aged 10–24 in developing regions (World Bank 1998). Pregnancy is the leading cause of death for young women aged 15–19 – complications from childbirth and unsafe abortions being the major factors (UNFPA 2003). Although less is known about young people's drug use in developing countries when compared with their sexual behaviour (UN 1997), we do know that poor young people – most especially those who live on the streets and those involved in sex work – are particularly vulnerable to the risks posed by drug use. In many cities across the world young people of 10 years old or less are using drugs (Deany 2000), using those substances that are cheapest and most readily available, such as glue and other inhalants. Research demonstrates that young people in a range of settings who feel frustrated by their limited economic options are more likely to engage in a range of risk behaviours, such as using drugs, unprotected sex and exchanging sex for gifts, money or favours (Rao Gupta, Whelan and Allendorf 2003).

Eaton, Flisher and Aaro (2003) have argued that sexual behaviour is influenced by factors operating at three levels: through *personal factors* – such as individual knowledge and beliefs, perception of risk and levels of self-esteem; through the *proximal context* – which refers to interpersonal relationships and the physical and organisational environment, for example relationships between genders, peers and with adults as well as access to media, to recreation and to contraception and condoms; and finally through the *distal context* – which refers to cultural and structural factors, such as the existence of patriarchy and broader social inequalities. However, upon careful examination it is clear that all of these levels are influenced in one way or another by poverty and inequalities. Looking at the South African context, the authors note that poverty, unemployment, overcrowding and low levels of education among young people are linked to both higher levels of sexual activity and less knowledge about sexual health. Poverty also leads to the commodification of sex, in addition to commercialised sex work, since for young women an older boyfriend or sexual partner may offer financial assistance that parents cannot. Socio-economic status is also related to the likelihood of young people experiencing physical and sexual coercion. The sexual domination of young women in particular is more common in poor communities (Eaton, Flisher and Aaro 2003). Poverty is highly implicated in homeless street life and the chances of being incarcerated in prison – two proximal contexts that hold elevated risk for HIV infection. Poor communities also have fewer recreational facilities for their young people and less access to the media, thereby increasing sexual activity and reducing access to information.

Young people who are concentrating on meeting their immediate economic needs, and facing daily threats to their health and well-being, such as those living on the streets, may be difficult to reach with messages about sexual health and illnesses or problems that may or may not affect them some time in the future (Aggleton and Rivers 1999). Unsurprisingly, young people who live and work on the streets of urban areas do not commonly list issues such as AIDS, hepatitis and STIs as over-riding concerns. Rather, the day-to-day need for shelter, food and clothes takes higher priority (Swart-Kruger and Richter 1997). Young poor people do not have the luxury of planning for their future – 'for the poor, it is the here and now that matters' (Cohen 2000: 2). Substance use problems disproportionately affect the most vulnerable – those who are poor and disenfranchised – from slum dwellers in New Delhi, hill tribes in northern Thailand to disadvantaged young people in central and Eastern Europe (Deany 2000).

As stated earlier, there is a clear relationship then between poverty and several of the recognised conditions that compound young people's social and health-related vulnerabilities. These include – but are not restricted to – lack of access to education, unequal gender roles, early childbearing, selling and exchanging sex, rural-to-urban migration and living on the streets, as well as mental and emotional health factors associated with economic and social inequality. Here each of these will be looked at in turn.

Access to education

It has been estimated that 115 million children do not attend primary school and that 57 million young men and 96 million young women aged 15–24 cannot read or write (UNICEF, UNAIDS and WHO 2002). Not surprisingly, these young people – the vast majority of whom live in the very poorest parts of the world – have less access to both employment and health information. As governments in poorer countries try to manage their burden of debt, and families struggle against poverty, schooling is often the sacrifice that has to be made – either because parents cannot afford the fees associated with schooling or because they need the children in the family to work.

However, education is widely acknowledged to reduce the chances of poor sexual and reproductive health and drug use. Young people with more years of schooling are less likely to have non-regular sexual partners and are more likely to use condoms than their peers with less schooling (UNAIDS 2003). Two thirds of those who do not attend school globally are girls – and girls in school are significantly less likely to have experienced sexual intercourse than girls who are not attending school (Finger, Lapetina and Pribila 2002). Education is known to increase girls' self-confidence, social and negotiation skills, as well as earning power – and this makes them less vulnerable to violence and sexual exploitation (UNICEF 2004)

Overall, not only is education in itself a protective factor in relation to sexual and reproductive health, it also provides a forum in which to deliver information and build skills in relationships. Out-of-school young people are harder to reach with health messages.

Gender roles

Gender inequalities are well recognised as a major factor driving poor sexual and reproductive health – and particularly the spread of HIV. However, there is also a clear relationship between gender inequality and poverty (Rivers and Aggleton 1999). First, girls and women are more likely to experience poverty than boys and men. Traditional ways of measuring poverty by looking at household income have sometimes obscured female poverty (Cagatay 1998). However, using measures of human poverty such as those suggested by UNDP (1997), the full extent of female poverty has been revealed. These measures show that there are many resources beyond income, such as education and health, which are unequally distributed between men and women – especially among those who are very poor. In poor households, resource allocation is often biased against girls and young women – for example, in terms of provision of the most nutritious food and purchasing health care and education – which may be more exclusively reserved for male children. There are also structural inequalities in the labour market, whereby women are excluded from certain jobs or paid less for the same or similar work as men. Much of young women's (and older women's) time may be used up in unpaid domestic labour and childcare – which does not generate income. And finally, women are more vulnerable to transient poverty – caused by familial, personal, social or economic crises – for example divorce and widowhood (Cagatay 1998).

Secondly, unequal gender roles may be reinforced and entrenched when people are living in poverty. Recent research in Mozambique, for example, has shown that schoolgirls from wealthier areas express a greater willingness to challenge stereotypical gender norms and report more assertive behaviour with boyfriends than young women in poorer suburbs, as well as fewer sexual partners and more frequent condom use (Machel 2001). Research in Tanzania (Seel 1996), Zimbabwe (Runganga and Aggleton 1998) and many other countries suggests that young men may attempt to address economic and inter-generational inequalities through sexual activity with multiple partners, which may be seen as symbolising advanced status and adulthood.

Poverty among girls and women, together with their overall economic dependence on men, also restricts their ability to make decisions about sex (Rivers and Aggleton 1999). Poorer young women often need the financial support of boyfriends and sexual partners – and so are less able to resist male domination. Young women's ability to demand condom use is compromised in conditions of poverty where boyfriends are often considered an important source of economic assistance (Campbell 2003: 128). Psychological factors linked to poverty may also discourage young women from challenging entrenched gender inequality: 'Young people, who have had little experience of ever having achieved important goals or life aspirations, may also feel disempowered to challenge stereotypical gender norms that place their sexual health at risk' (Campbell 2003: 184).

Drug-related behaviour is also highly gendered, with young men being more at risk of substance abuse than young women. Poor people across the world report that alcohol and drug use are major consequences of poverty among male family members (WHO/WB 2002). In Eastern Europe and central Asia, injecting drugs has become widespread among young men. In countries across central Asia, the Russian Federation and central and Eastern Europe, it is estimated that 70 per cent of people injecting drugs are under 25. Half of the people injecting drugs are aged 16–25 years (UNICEF, UNAIDS and WHO 2002).

Drug dependency increases the likelihood that some young people will turn to crime and sex work in order to finance their drug habit (UNICEF, UNAIDS and WHO 2002). Ideologies of masculinity that emphasise risk taking as well as the need for material success, drive some poor young men to become involved in drug production and trafficking – and to use substances themselves to bolster low self-esteem caused by conditions of poverty. In addition to the risks associated with drug use (particularly injecting drug use), young people's reported alcohol and drug risk behaviours are often strongly correlated with having unsafe sex (Finger, Lapetina and Pribila 2002).

Early childbearing

Although early marriage – and subsequent early childbearing – occurs in many parts of the world, poverty exerts a pressure on families to marry girls early in order to have one less mouth to feed. Mikhail (2002) has argued that 'child' marriage is most often precipitated by economic vulnerability linked to limited life options, and it is significant that early marriage is most common in parts of Africa and south Asia. In Niger, 76 per cent of girls are married by the age of 18, while in India the figure is 50 per cent. In Nepal, 19 per cent of girls are married by the age of 15, with 60 per cent being married by age 18 (UNICEF, UNAIDS and WHO 2002). Early marriage and childbearing contribute to high maternal mortality. Globally, those aged 15–19 years are twice as likely as women in their twenties to die in childbirth (UNFPA 2003). Poverty and unequal power relations make it hard for girls to resist the pressure to marry early to a partner of their family's choice, and in many countries young women are married to much older, more sexually experienced men, which may place them at risk of STIs and HIV.

The level of family poverty is strongly correlated with earlier sexual debut for girls even in settings where early marriage is not the norm (Finger, Lapetina and Pribila 2002). Poor young unmarried women are more likely than older women to have clandestine or illegal abortions. When young women do go ahead with pregnancy, early motherhood can cut short a girl's education – another factor related to poor sexual and reproductive health, and increasing poverty (Finger, Lapetina and Pribila 2002).

Selling and exchanging sex

Sex work is an area in which the relationship between poverty and risk behaviour is radically apparent. The international trafficking in women and girls is a feature of global poverty and unemployment (Shifman 2003). Children and young people – especially girls – are particularly vulnerable to being sold into the sex trade. It has been estimated that one million children are abducted or coerced into the sex trade each year (UNICEF, UNAIDS and WHO 2002). In Nepal, for example, trafficking of Nepalese girls and young women is an integral part of the social and economic fabric (Poudel and Carryer 2000). Along with suffering and degradation, this places the young women at high risk of poor mental, physical and sexual and reproductive health.

In addition to young people who are trafficked this way, poverty tends to lead generally to the increasing commodification – and commercialisation –

of sex (Eaton, Flisher and Aaro 2003). Campbell (2003) has conducted research among mining communities in South Africa and reports on a thriving commercial sex industry. She writes that 'in women's accounts of how they had become sex workers, a number of common themes emerged, including the death of spouses or parents, dropping out of school after falling pregnant, and finding it difficult to find work, leaving an abusive man, or "running away" from the poverty and hardships of home' (Campbell 2003: 64).

In addition to being a driver for selling and exchanging sex, poverty also mitigates against the practice of safe sex among sex workers. Bhave *et al.* (1995), in a study in Mumbai, found that although sex workers may want to practise safe sex, they face losing a considerable amount of money by doing so – so that fear of loss of income is one of the most important factors in deterring sex workers from using condoms. As Ntsoakae Phatlane (2003: 83) has put it, writing about South Africa, 'Poverty plays a critical role in that it limits . . . bargaining power, as a result of which many [sex workers] . . . are compelled to put themselves at risk in order to satisfy their clients by yielding to demands for unprotected sex.'

Even where poor young people are not involved in selling sex, exchanging sex for survival is common. Research in Namibia – where about 60 per cent of the population live on less than US$2 a day – has shown that young women and single mothers in poverty were most likely to have sex with wage earners in employment (Mufune 2003). In one of the poorest regions of Namibia – Eenhara – those worst hit by poverty had high levels of alcohol consumption, and also reported exchanging sex for alcohol (Mufune 2003). In this context and in others, girls and women are often forced by poverty into multiple sexual relationships in order to increase their chances of getting food, clothes and education (Ntsoakae Phatlane 2003).

Rural to urban migration

The growth of a poor urban population as a result of dramatic rural–urban migration across the globe in the last forty years has resulted in increasing numbers of poor urban young people (Esim *et al.* 2001). Migration affects sexual health in a number of ways (see also chapter 10). First, people who migrate for work usually do so without their conjugal partners – leaving the migrant worker vulnerable to buying sex in urban or other work settings; secondly, men in particular are often removed from the family home and are no longer involved in the socialisation of children and young people, destabilising the family; and thirdly, young people themselves are encouraged through poverty to seek employment away from the influence of their family and may set up residence many miles away from the usual forms of support. In many parts of the world, traditional multi-generational extended families are increasingly being replaced with nuclear families, lone-parent families and the absence of parents or adult support (Aggleton and Rivers 1999).

Ntsoakae Phatlane (2003) has examined the role that apartheid-created poverty has played in fuelling and driving the HIV epidemic in South Africa. Under apartheid, Bantustans (rural homelands) served as 'dumping grounds' for those not needed by the white economy – the elderly, the sick, children and those caring for them. Adult males were forced into migrant labour, which placed them in often precarious work environments such as mining. This simultaneously undermined conjugal stability and long-term monogamous relationships as well as the role of the father in the family (Ntsoakae Phatlane 2003). Male migrant workers meanwhile – alone and often engaged in arduous and dangerous work – used alcohol and sex workers to achieve some escape from their circumstances, leading to STIs and HIV infection, which many of them unwittingly took back to the Bantustans to their wives.

Clearly, it is not only poor adults who are forced to migrate from home to seek work. As a result of familial poverty, there are millions of young people who are employed in cities in domestic service and other low paid jobs, which remove them from their families and place them at risk of sexual abuse and exploitation (Esim *et al.* 2001). Without adult support and protection – as well as love or companionship – young people are vulnerable not only to sexual exploitation, but also to early sexual relationships with peers.

Living and working on the streets

Across the world, millions of young people eke out a living on city streets, where they may survive by trading or selling sex – but are also extremely vulnerable to rape and sexual exploitation (UNAIDS 2003). An estimated 10,000 children live or work on the streets of South Africa; while the three Indian cities of Calcutta, Delhi and Mumbai are home to at least 100,000 street children. Many of these children exchange sex for money, goods or protection: more than half of the street children interviewed in a South African study reported making such exchanges (Swart-Kruger and Richter 1997). Street children in Jakarta, Indonesia have reported that being forced to have sex is one of the greatest problems that they face (Black and Farrington 1997).

Research conducted with street boys aged between 9 and 23 years in Bangalore, India revealed that the most common explanation offered for leaving home was poverty (Ramakrishna *et al.* 2004). Older boys often sought sexual favours from younger boys in return for protection – 44 per cent of interviewees said they had been sexually abused and most were sexually active before their teens. In addition, street boys displayed very high rates of use of alcohol and drugs, including solvents and marijuana.

While they recognised some of the risks of their lifestyle, and knew that condoms could protect them, they commented that they were 'not in a position to make decisions regarding the adoption of safer sexual practices' (Ramakrishna *et al.* 2004: 67).

In Tanzania, where poor families are under considerable pressure, an increasing number of boys and girls are living independently on the streets of towns and cities. These street children, some of whom have been orphaned as a result of AIDS, have been subjected to exploitation and rejection by their extended families, and are exposed to considerable risks of abuse, sexual violence and HIV within the street environment (Evans 2002).

Mental and emotional health

Not surprisingly, poverty – and the survival strategies that poor people sometimes have to cope with – have psychological implications. Mental health problems, such as stress, anxiety, depression and lack of self-esteem, were among the effects of poverty commonly identified by poor people in every region of the world.

In Eastern Europe and central Asia, in particular, the onset of sudden poverty is widely reported as leading to psychological problems (WHO/WB 2002). Rigi (2003) has described how the increase in socio-economic inequalities since the demise of Soviet communism in Kazakhstan has affected young people. He argues that neo-liberal reforms along with a rise in consumerism have transformed the conditions of youth. Post-Soviet Kazakhstan has seen the rise of an élite wealthy majority, while the majority of the population – in the absence of access to education and secure jobs that they formerly had – have sunk into dire poverty. Although Soviet society was clearly stratified, with the children of influential parents enjoying material advantages and access to the best university places and job opportunities, other young people did have basic rights, including education, jobs and sports and cultural resources. In the post-Soviet era, polarisation between rich and poor has increased. Poor young people in particular have been pushed towards deviant economic activities – such as crime and sex work.

Rigi (2003) interviewed young people and found that poor youth have an acute sense of deprivation and are gloomy about their future. While young people share a consumerist mentality, the reality of their prospects has led young people to deal with the present through sex and drugs. In this context, 'sexual promiscuity is a source of adventure and fun' – with sexual activity usually beginning for girls and boys from the age of 13 (Rigi 2003: 43). Many socially excluded young men have become widely involved in gangs engaging in petty theft, minor racketeering and drug dealing, while poor young women have resorted to exchanging and selling sex.

The rapid growth of drug use and drug injecting since 1990 in Eastern and central Europe is well known, and largely thought to be a result of dramatic unemployment, increased income differentials and poverty (Deany 2000). In the year 2000 in Russia, there was twenty times more drug use reported than in 1990, with an estimated 700,000 drug users nationally (Deany 2000).

In poor communities, chronic unemployment and the limitation of job options to low skills, low wage positions frustrate and humiliate young men still taught to see themselves as economic providers: 'endemic poverty breeds fatalism and deep-seated anger that may encourage both personal risk-taking and indifference to others' (Irwin, Millen and Fallows 2003: 24). This in turn impacts upon gender relations, increasing sexual and physical violence towards women.

Conclusions

Many of those working in development, sexual and reproductive health and substance use acknowledge that initiatives to change sexual behaviour and substance use among poor people are unlikely to be successful, unless the root causes – including poverty and stark economic inequalities, as well as gender inequalities – are addressed. As Berer (2003: 9–10) has put it,

> The role of macro socio-economic conditions in fostering unsafe sexual relationships also deserves greater attention. . . . These include the lack of decently paid work for the great majority of women in most developing countries, especially the poorest; employment and migration policies that force large numbers of men and women to migrate for work leaving behind their spouses and families; and tourism and drug dealing that are tied to the sex industry . . . the commercialisation and commodification of sex, the proliferation of trading and selling sex for money and goods, and of multiple partnering, casual sex and frequent partner change. Reducing these conditions would be far more effective in promoting sexual health at a population level than only trying to change the sexual behaviour of millions of individuals one by one.

However, despite such understanding sexual and reproductive health and substance programmes continue to use strategies designed to bring about individual behaviour change with little regard for the structural factors that constrain people's choices and inhibit safer practices. Writing particularly in relation to AIDS, Irwin, Millen and Fallows (2003: 20) argue that:

> The myth that people contract AIDS because they refuse to make 'lifestyle changes' is based on a belief that everyone can select from the same menu of options. The daily lives of affluent, educated people in wealthy countries do provide numerous opportunities to make choices . . . [but when] this model of personal choice . . . [is] projected into contexts of poverty . . . [it distorts our view] . . . The language of sexual

or lifestyle choice exaggerates the degree of agency that many people are able to exercise.

They continue:

> the most powerful factor restricting people's abilities to make sound choices about sexual practices and substance use is poverty. In combination with other social factors – above all inequality in the distribution of wealth and social power – poverty limits people's options from protecting themselves and forces them into situations of heightened risk.
>
> (Irwin, Millen and Fallows 2003: 21)

In summary, poor young people – great numbers of whom live in developing countries – are particularly vulnerable to sexual and drug-related ill-health. Even where young people do not live in absolute poverty, but are among those disadvantaged by vast disparities between rich and poor, the impact on sexual and drug-related health is clear to see. Not only do young people have less economic opportunity than older people, but they also have fewer rights and less power than adults. This can lead to frustration and may cause some young people to seek adult status in ways that are injurious to their health. The most vulnerable of all young people are young women and young people from minority ethnic groups, who usually have the least access to economic and other resources, such as information, education and health care. Policy makers and those working with young people at a programmatic level need to acknowledge the influence and impact of poverty on young people's lives if strides are to be made in improving sexual health and managing substance-related harms.

For development to occur, economic growth must be accompanied by efforts to tackle inequalities. While economic growth is known to reduce absolute poverty, unless it is human-centred, it may increase disparities between the rich and the poor. Development agencies and governments need to work together closely to ensure that the benefits of economic growth are more equally shared. This may mean that new forms of regulation will be required in the world economy in order to help achieve greater equality, alongside the promotion of human rights.

Programmes that do not take into account the reality of young people's lives will have little impact on sexual health and substance use. Some programmes to promote sexual health and reduce substance-related harm have attempted to promote livelihood skills among young people. Such work has not been adequately explored or evaluated to date (Esim et al. 2001) and it is important that such programmes are developed and evaluated, so that they might be more widely adopted.

As well as taking young people's economic realities into account, programmes need to take account of their perceived needs. Research has shown that young people are often frustrated by their lack of economic and social power and by the inequalities they see around them. This, in turn, can impact upon the choices they make about sexual and drug-related behaviour. These issues need to be more fully explored in future work. Programmes for young women, in particular, need to take account of the triple jeopardy of youth, poverty and gender. Young women clearly have fewer economic opportunities and less social power. Programmes for boys too need to encourage more equitable gender norms.

References

Aggleton, P. and Rivers, K. (1999) 'Interventions for Adolescents', in L. Gibney, R.J. DiClemente and S.H. Vermund (eds) *Preventing HIV in Developing Countries*, New York: Plenum.

Berer, M. (2003) 'HIV/AIDS, Sexual and Reproductive Health: Intimately Related', *Reproductive Health Matters*, 11 (22): 6–11.

Bhave, G., Lindan, C.P., Hudes, E.S., Desia, S., Wagle, U., Tripathi, S.P. and Mandel, J.S. (1995) 'Impact of and Intervention on HIV, Sexually Transmitted Diseases, and Condom Use Among Sex Workers in Bombay, India', *AIDS*, 9 (Suppl. 1): S21–S30.

Black, B. and Farrington, A.P. (1997) 'Preventing HIV/AIDS by Promoting Life for Indonesian Street Children', *AIDS Captions*, 4: 14–17.

Burns, A.A., Daileader Rutland, C. and Finger, W. with Murphy-Graham, E., McCarney, R. and Schueller, J. (2004) *Reaching Out-of-School Youth with Reproductive Health and HIV/AIDS Information and Services*, Arlington, VA: Family Health International.

Cagatay, N. (1998) *Gender and Poverty*, New York: UNDP.

Campbell, C. (2003) *Letting Them Die*, Wetton, South Africa: Double Storey.

Chronic Poverty Research Centre (2002) *Chronic Poverty Update*, July 2002. Online. Available HTTP: <www.chronicpoverty.org>

Cohen, D. (2000) *Poverty and HIV/AIDS in Sub-Saharan Africa*, New York: UNDP.

Deany, P. (2000) *HIV and Injecting Drug Use: A New Challenge to Sustainable Human Development*, Bangkok: UNDP South-East Asia HIV and Development Program.

Eaton, L., Flisher, A.J. and Aaro, L.E. (2003) 'Unsafe Sexual Behaviour in South African Youth', *Social Science and Medicine*, 56: 149–65.

Esim, S. and Malhotra, A., Mathur, S., Duron, G. and Johnson-Welch, C. (2001) *Making it Work: Linking Youth, Reproductive Health and Livelihoods*, Washington, DC: International Center for Research on Women.

Evans, R. (2002) 'Poverty, HIV and Barriers to Education: Street Children's Experiences in Tanzania', *Gender and Development*, 10: 51–62.

Finger, B., Lapetina, M. and Pribila, M. (eds) (2002) *Intervention Strategies that Work for Youth*, Arlington, VA: Family Health International.

Irwin, A., Millen, J. and Fallows, D. (2003) *Global AIDS: Myths and Facts: Tools for Fighting the AIDS Pandemic*, Cambridge, MA: South End Press.

Jana, S., Bandyopadhay, N., Dutta, M.K. and Sana, A. (2002) 'A Tale of Two Cities:

Shifting the Paradigm of Anti-Trafficking Programmes', *Gender and Development*, 10: 69–79.

Machel, J. (2001) 'Unsafe Sexual Behaviour Amongst Schoolgirls in Mozambique: A Matter of Gender and Class', *Reproductive Health Matters*, 9: 82–92.

Maclean, A. (1999) *Sewing for a Better Future? Discussions with Young Garment Factory Workers in Cambodia about Life, Work and Sexual Health*, Washington, DC: Care International.

Mikhail, S.L.B. (2002) 'Child Marriage and Prostitution: Two Forms of Sexual Exploitation?' *Gender and Development*, 10: 43–9.

Mufune, P. (2003) 'Changing Patterns of Sexuality in Northern Namibia: Implications for the Transmission of HIV/AIDS', *Culture, Health and Sexuality*, 5: 425–38.

Ntsoakae Phatlane, S. (2003) 'Poverty and HIV/AIDS in Apartheid South Africa', *Social Identities*, 9: 73–91.

Population Council (2002) *Youth and HIV/AIDS*, New York: Population Council.

Poudel, P. and Carryer, J. (2000) 'Girl-trafficking, HIV/AIDS, and the Position of Women in Nepal', *Gender and Development*, 8: 74–9.

Ramakrishna, J., Karott, M., Murthy, R.S., Chandran, V. and Pelto, P.J. (2004) 'Sexual Behaviours of Street Boys and Male Sex Workers in Bangalore', in R.K. Verma, P.J. Pelto, S.L. Schensul and A. Joshi (eds) *Sexuality in the Time of AIDS*, New Delhi: Sage.

Rao Gupta, G., Whelan, D. and Allendorf, K. (2003) *Integrating Gender into HIV/AIDS Programmes*, Geneva: UNAIDS.

Rigi, J. (2003) 'The Conditions of Post-Soviet Dispossessed Youth and Work in Almaty, Kazakhstan', *Critique of Anthropology*, 23: 35–49.

Rivers, K. and Aggleton, P. (1999) *Men and the HIV Epidemic*, New York: UNDP.

Runganga, A. and Aggleton, P. (1998) 'Migration, the Family and the Transformation of a Sexual Culture', *Sexualities*, 1: 63–81.

Seel, P. (1996) 'AIDS as a Paradox of Manhood and Development in Kilimanjaro, Tanzania', *Social Science and Medicine*, 43: 1169–78.

Shifman, P. (2003) 'Trafficking and Women's Human Rights in a Globalised World', *Gender and Development*, 11: 125–32.

Swart-Kruger, J. and Richter, L.M. (1997) 'AIDS-Related Knowledge, Attitudes and Behaviour among South African Street Youth: Reflections on Power, Sexuality and the Autonomous Self', *Social Science and Medicine*, 45: 957–66.

UN (1997) *Statement of Commitment: United Nations Commission on Sustainable Development*, Overall Review and Appraisal of the Implementation of Agenda 21, Report of the 7th Session.

UN (1999) *Youth and Drugs: A Global Overview*, Geneva: United Nations.

UNAIDS (2003) *HIV/AIDS and Young People – Hope for Tomorrow*, Geneva: UNAIDS.

UNAIDS/WHO (2001) *AIDS Epidemic Update*, Geneva: UNAIDS/WHO.

UNDP (1997) *Human Development Report 1997*, New York: Oxford University Press.

UNFPA (2003) *Achieving the Millennium Development Goals*, New York: UNFPA.

UNICEF (2004) *The State of the World's Children*, New York: UNICEF.

UNICEF, UNAIDS and WHO (2002) *Young People and HIV/AIDS: Opportunity in Crisis*, New York: UNICEF.

World Bank (1998) *Investing in Young Lives: The Role of Reproductive Health*, Washington, DC: World Bank.

World Health Organization (WHO) (1998) *Coming of Age: From Facts to Action for Adolescent Sexual and Reproductive Health*, Geneva: WHO.

WHO/WB (2002) *Dying for Change: Poor People's Experience of Health and Ill-Health*, Geneva: WHO/WB.

Chapter 3

Gender, vulnerability and young people

Rita M. Melendez and Deborah L. Tolman

Forming and enjoying sexual relations is a normal part of human development. However, sex is also an arena in which a number of health-related vulnerabilities can and do occur, and these vulnerabilities are patterned depending on whether one is female or male. This chapter aims to describe the gender dimensions of some of the health-related vulnerabilities that young people may experience. Two broad sets of factors contribute to detrimental sexual health outcomes such as HIV infection – individual risk and societal vulnerability (Mane and Aggleton 2001). Individual risk is characterized by what individuals know and how they choose to act to reduce or increase their risk. Societal vulnerability, on the other hand, stems from socio-cultural, economic, legal and political factors that limit individuals' options to reduce their risk. Although the two are interrelated, gender is a key to both individual risk and societal vulnerability.

We will begin by presenting two examples of young women, Renu and Janet, with different sexual health risks, exemplifying the differences between individual risk and societal vulnerabilities. This is followed by an overview of gender and patriarchy, examining how gender affects health outcomes, including specific examples of how gender is incorporated and enacted within both social structures and by individuals. We then look more closely at these processes by examining the broad and interrelating areas of poverty, violence and legal rights. Finally, we offer three case studies to demonstrate different ways in which young persons' vulnerability can be reduced through gender-based programmes and interventions.

Renu is 15 years old and lives in rural Nepal.[1] Her family lives in extreme poverty and struggles to survive. Renu feels obligated to contribute to her family's subsistence, even though she is unable, by law, to inherit any of her family's property. She knows many other girls her age who have left their homes to earn money for the family, and offers to travel to the Nepali capital, Katmandu, to search for work and to send money to her family, which, in her community, is not outside of the norm.

In Katmandu, Renu is alone in an unfamiliar place. Frightened, she has no one to talk to; hoping to find work, she does not know where to begin to look. She is approached by a man offering her a job with 'good pay' and 'under good conditions'. Being completely isolated, there is no one to tell her what they know about this man and think about his offer. Feeling she has no other options, she accepts. She is sent to Mumbai, beaten and forced to work in a brothel. Her attempts to escape the brothel are only met with more beatings and electric shocks. She has to service many men and most refuse to wear condoms; Renu soon contracts HIV.

Despite these hardships, Renu is lucky. Unlike many Nepali women taken to India for forced sex work, Renu is rescued by Indian police. Although the rescue was pivotal for Renu, at the same time it produced a new set of problems. Both the Indian and Nepali governments refuse to pay for Renu's and other young women's voyage back to Nepal. Again by luck, Nepali charity organizations discover Renu's plight and pay for her trip back to her village. Now Renu wants to warn other young women in her village about the dangers she experienced.

Janet is a 15-year-old White girl who lives in a middle-class, suburban neighbourhood in the USA. She is not rich, but she does not have to worry about any basic, material needs – her parents take care of those for her. Janet wants to be liked by her friends and the boys at school. It has not been hard for her to work out that girls at school who have boyfriends are considered prettier and more popular than girls without boyfriends. Janet

---

1 This account is based in part on the true story reported by Ganga Gurung (1998).

is happy she has a boyfriend and even happier he is older than the other girls' boyfriends. Martin is in his first year of college. He likes Janet because she is young. He likes that he can tell Janet what to do and that she doesn't argue with him, like some girls of his own age.

Janet and Martin have been going out for a few months. Both of them think it is a good relationship. Martin occasionally calls Janet 'stupid' or a 'slut' so she will change how she acts and dresses. When he gets angry, he throws things at Janet and pushes her. Since he is older, Martin feels like he needs to teach Janet how to act and believes that he only does these things for Janet's own good. Although Janet is hurt by his insults and behaviour, she knows that many other girls' boyfriends also call them names and push them around. She is happy to be together with Martin and accepts his actions as part of who he is. She thinks he will change in the future.

Janet and Martin have been having sex for a while now. It was not something Janet had planned to do, 'it just happened', as so many girls her age report. Partly, she did not resist Martin because she knew how much he wanted to be with her and she didn't want to lose him. Janet doesn't really feel anything when she has sex. When others talk about how great sex is, Janet goes along with them, but she doesn't really know what they're talking about. She is worried about getting pregnant or even getting a sexually transmitted infection, but she has no one to talk to about safer sex or contraception. The only time her parents talk to her about sex is when they are telling her not to have sex with Martin, and she worries that if she asks someone else, they will think she is a 'slut' . . .

While Renu and Janet's lives could not be more different in many ways, there are similarities that may not be immediately evident. Both of these stories are about the choices that are available to girls in the places where they are growing up, as well as how these choices are limited by economic and social circumstances. The ways that relationships play a very significant role in girls' risk and ability to make safe choices, and the consequences of limited information about what girls should and should not expect or accept from men and boys are illuminated. Both of these stories are about how gender – behaviour and expectations about being a girl/woman and also being a boy/man – is a key structural element in girls' sexuality. Both of these stories show how individual girls live in overlapping circles of contexts – relationships, economics, social expectations and norms, availability of resources and information – that are an inextricable part of girls' ability to make choices.

Vulnerability

Youth and adolescence are periods of life that offer opportunities and limitations. In many, if not most societies, the transition into adulthood is marked by life-changing events and decisions that can place young people at risk of detrimental health outcomes. The contextual circumstances in which young people develop – community, family, economic, religious, political and social norms that include the possibilities and limits due to gender and age – have a great deal to do with how individuals negotiate or even are aware of such risks. The contexts of Renu and Janet's lives, although very different, left them both vulnerable. Health-related vulnerability means exposure to violence, drug use, sexually transmitted infections, HIV, unwanted pregnancies and general lack of health care, outcomes that negatively affect both the psychological and physical health of individuals and that severely limit an individual's life choices.

While Renu and Janet's stories highlight the perspective of individuals, the choices and experiences of individuals have a broader impact. Collectively, negative health outcomes can break down social and cultural systems in society and limit a country's economic development (Upton 2003). Understanding the processes of sexual vulnerability in young people's lives has far-reaching implications for improving the health of both individuals and societies.

Gender

Gender is a key factor shaping young people's lives and vulnerabilities. The basis of the distinction between women and men is a presumption of male and female anatomy; however, gender is principally about the behaviours, thoughts and emotions, and their expression, associated with 'appropriate' male and female characteristics (Connell 1999). We are given gendered meanings – how to act as a man or a woman – that are inscribed in customs, laws and traditions. Gender works together with larger social, cultural and economic structures to limit resources, ensuring that some individuals are more vulnerable to health risks than others. How individuals enact gender, as well as the structural barriers surrounding gender, limit access to health-related resources and may result in detrimental health outcomes (Amaro 1995).

The varied uses of 'gender' reflect a number of different and contested theories (Tolman *et al.* 2003b), including evolutionary theory, in which gender is grounded in biological or physical characteristics that have historically separated male and female behaviour (Buss 1999); social role theory, in which gender is understood in terms of norms or roles that differentiate masculine and feminine qualities and behaviour (Pleck 1987; Spence 1993); and social construction theory, in which gender is understood as a set of practices and performances constituted through language or discourses and 'performance' (Butler 1993) and a feature of a pervasive yet invisible political system constituted through society's institutions (Connell 1995).

A social constructionist approach yields insight into the processes by which gender shapes various dimensions of young people's lives. For some writers and practitioners, the concept of 'doing gender' has become a useful one in understanding gender from the social constructionist perspective. As West and Zimmerman (1987) explain, gender is both a cultural construct and a feature of the social structure, perpetuated because we are continually 'doing gender'. That is, by engaging in the process of behaving in, thinking about, or even feeling in the prescribed ways that our society ascribes to males and females, each person actively enacts gender – over and over and over again. This process makes it virtually impossible to 'see' the production of gender until one is aware of this process. Thus, gender relations, as well as gendered individuals, are constantly created, maintained and reproduced in everyday life. From this theoretical perspective, people do not act out preordained or hard-wired gender categories; rather, people are effective in creating gender in their everyday actions and interactions with others.

However, gender is not a purely individual process. People learn how to do gender from cultural norms and through socialization experiences. How we do gender is constrained and constructed by larger social institutions and processes. For example, gender is dependent upon the individual characteristics of race, class and education (West and Fenstermaker 1995). At the same time, gender is also dependent on the larger political and social processes such as political systems, poverty and immigration. That is, gender is never constructed in a vacuum but is also always informed by other individual and social structures; for instance, the life of a young, poor boy living in a developing country will be completely different from a college-aged young man living in the USA, yet there are likely to be some commonalities associated with the fact that they are both males in their societies.

While each individual makes some choices about how to enact gender, including each person's definition of themselves as male or female, these choices are always contextualized by how a society or community ascribes appropriate gender behaviour and self concepts to men and women. Individuals can make choices about how to be male or female, but when going against the grain of societal expectations there are often consequences that are social, economic or even physical. However, staying within gender boundaries can also, as the cases of Renu and Janet underscore, make an individual vulnerable. Gender is one way, among many, to marginalize people, to exclude them from needed resources and to take away their human rights.

Women: 'doing gender' within structure

How does gender affect the lives of young women? And more importantly how does gender create and contribute to health-related vulnerabilities? There is general consent that women are in a position of less power vis-à-vis men in virtually all societies. Many theorists point to patriarchy to understand unequal power distributions in society. Broadly speaking, patriarchy is a system in which men are in charge of the family and where the family organization is reflected in larger social structures. In most societies, men tend to control institutions such as government and the economy, as well as culture and civil society. Wealth, both material wealth and cultural wealth, is passed from father to son. Men are educated to take on positions of power and to carry on with the traditions they have learned (Scott 1999).

Patriarchy results in a number of health-related vulnerabilities for young women. Eight characteristics of patriarchy lead directly or indirectly to debilitating health outcomes such as violence and unwanted pregnancies (Gough 1975; Rich 1999).

1 Denying women their sexuality as with female genital cutting, chastity belts and denying women sexual information and services.
2 Forcing male sexuality upon women, for example, rape, domestic violence, incest, forced marriage and idealization of sexual violence in pornography.
3 Exploiting women's labour as in the segregation of women in low paid jobs and the denial of contraception and abortion that prevent women from choosing if and when they want children.
4 Robbing women of their children, as seen in laws granting fathers the right to take their children from their mothers and the enforced sterilization of women.
5 Confining women physically and preventing their movement by means of rape as a form of terror that often compels women to stay at home, sexual harassment on the streets and at work and cultural norms suggesting women stay at home.
6 Using women as objects in male transactions, for example in the sex slave trade, pimping and forced marriage.
7 Restricting women's creativeness through obstructing women's access to education and life outside the home and by defining male pursuits as 'more valuable' than female pursuits.
8 Preventing women from accessing large areas of society's knowledge and culture as seen in the lack of educational opportunities for women and their inability to live life without the supervision of fathers, brothers or husbands.

The marginalization and denigration of anything considered 'feminine' or passive also has the effect of 'tainting' anything or anybody who appears or behaves in ways that can be categorized as feminine. Thus, young men who violate norms of masculinity can often experience gender as a form of vulnerability, especially as it intersects with poverty, age and education.

Although Gough and Rich examine how male power creates women's vulnerabilities, it is important to remember that patriarchy is a complex system that involves larger global, political and social processes – both men and women contribute to and resist this system. Bringing together structure and individual ways of being, women are often in situations where they are forced to stay in positions of vulnerability or even to enter into positions where they realize they will be vulnerable. Renu and Janet each had different concerns. Renu was worried about getting money to take care of her family. Janet was worried about being liked and having a boyfriend. For each of these girls, these worries were at the heart of their sexual health choices. Although both these young women came from very different backgrounds, gender was a large factor in formulating their life experiences, futures and negative health outcomes. Renu acted out what others expected from her as a young woman. Her enactment of gender was structured by poverty, immigration, and the sex trafficking industry. The result of Renu's migration was violence and HIV infection. While Janet did not live in a world of extreme poverty or experience migration, she too enacted gender in a manner that was consistent with her situation and detrimental to her health. Janet's difficulty in wanting, knowing about or asking for contraception or safer sex, her acceptance of relationship violence as an expected part of having a boyfriend, and her limited access to information about sexuality are structured by cultural norms and social consequences that regulate her comfort and control over her sexuality.

It is important to recognize that young men too are vulnerable to the detrimental sexual health effects of patriarchy. Men are expected to uphold the characteristics of masculinity often encouraging them to engage in sex with many different partners. Where women are expected to be ignorant and passive with regards to sexual relationships, men are expected to be knowledgeable and active. Dominant norms of masculinity may prevent some young men from seeking information and admitting that they may lack pertinent sexual information (Rao Gupta 2000). Additionally, the emphasis on male sexual 'experience' may oblige men to have sex with as many different partners as possible, thereby increasing their exposure to sexually transmitted infections. Research suggests that HIV-related risks (for both men and women) are greater when women are expected to please men and to defer to their authority (UNAIDS 1999).

Poverty and gender

Young men and women are disproportionately affected by poverty, as are women in general (Bianchi 1999). Poverty exacerbates the effects of patriarchy for both women and men. Furthermore, it establishes a foundation on which a number of sexual health concerns emerge for both young women and men. According to the United Nations (UNAIDS 2003), worldwide, women earn slightly more than 50 per cent of what men earn and the majority of the 1.3 billion people living on one dollar a day or less are women and children.

Over the years, globalization has had a huge and often detrimental effect on the health of young women. Throughout Asia, Africa and Latin America, large numbers of women work in factories for small wages and no benefits. These factories often lack safety precautions and can have adverse consequences on women's health (Pearson 1994). Employers in such factories cite the need for female physical qualities (e.g. women have more 'nimble fingers' than men) as a reason for hiring a majority of women (Pearson 1998). In some situations, women may be more able to find work and support their families than are men. This situation too can result in violence against women, as it constitutes an often profound violation of social expectations that men provide for their families, leading to shame, humiliation and anger among men that often finds expression in violence that is (mis)directed at women (England and Farkas 1986). Research in some countries demonstrates that men who are unemployed often feel they have lost their status as providers and may be more likely to have sex with sex workers or other partners to regain their sense of masculinity (UNAIDS 2003).

War and political instability interact with poverty to further impact upon young people's health. Young women suffer an immediate impact of such conflicts, including state-sponsored violence, loss of income, and displacement. At the same time, women must try to provide for and protect their families, as well as themselves, from starvation, bodily harm and disease. As a result of war and political instability, there were 25 million refugees in the world in 1996. The majority of refugees are women and children. Displacement causes health problems related to the inaccessibility of health care for pregnancies and child birth, resulting in increased rates of perinatal mortality and congenital abnormalities (Carballo and Simic 1996). Likewise, war and political instability also negatively affect the lives of young men who are often forced to engage in battle or to move, leaving their families, in search of paid labour. The instability caused by poverty often leaves young men without familiar foundations and unable to contribute to their households. Several research studies have demonstrated that men in the military have higher rates of HIV; partly, this increased risk is explained by increased sexual activity while away from home (see also chapter 11) (UNAIDS 2003).

Violence and gender

Gender-based violence takes many forms. Around the world, one in three women report experiencing violence by an intimate partner (Heise and Elias

1995). In the USA, a national probability survey conducted in 1998 found that one out of every four women has been physically abused and/or raped by an intimate partner. Of women who reported they had been raped, 22 per cent were under age 12 when they were first raped, and 32 per cent were between 12 and 17 years of age (Tjaden and Thoennes 2000). A recent study in New Zealand found that among women aged 20 to 22, 25 per cent of those who had had sexual intercourse before age 14 reported that their first intercourse occasion had been forced (Dickson *et al.* 1998). In another study conducted in Jamaica, 40 per cent of girls aged 11–15 reported that their first sexual intercourse had been forced (Allen 1982). Many sexual abuse survivors experience shame and stigma. Many feel vulnerable, unloved and unable to say 'no' to things they do not want to do, such as having sex or using drugs.

The patterns for violence in intimate relationships may begin in the early years of young people's development. The pervasiveness of sexual harassment, for example, is well documented in secondary schools. About 80 per cent of young women in secondary schools reported that they have been victims of sexual harassment, naming both verbal and physical abuse from boys (AAUW 1993; HRW 2001; Lee *et al.* 1996; Stein 1999). There may be a slippery slope from the normalized incidents of sexual harassment that occur in school to violence in simultaneously occurring early dating experiences. Sexual harassment in schools may inadvertently function as a kind of dress rehearsal for heterosexual relationships more generally (Tolman *et al.* 2003a).

Many researchers have noted the clear association between violence in sexual relationships and the prevalence of HIV. A large proportion of men and women who are HIV-positive report experiences of abuse (Cohen *et al.* 2000). In the USA, people who reported being raped as a child were more likely to have engaged in sex work and risky sexual behaviours than people who did not report childhood sexual violence (Wingood and DiClemente 1997). Men and women who have experienced abuse as a child often find themselves in a cycle of abuse that repeats itself throughout their lives (Browne 1993). Research on women who have experienced partner abuse shows they are more likely than other women to experience depression, anxiety, substance abuse, suicidal ideation and suicide attempts (Browne 1993). Abused women report lower perceptions of control over safer sex and lower self-efficacy in negotiating safer sex with their partners (Beadnell *et al.* 2000). Additionally, many abused women fear violence on the part of their partner when negotiating safer sex (Kalichman *et al.* 1998) and are more likely to incur abuse as a result of requesting a partner to use a condom (Wingood and DiClemente 1997).

Legal rights and gender

The lack of legal rights for girls and women may be a precursor for poverty and violence. According to the UNAIDS-led *Global Coalition on Women and AIDS*, where women lack the ability to own property including land, they suffer increased poverty, violence and reduced personal security (UNAIDS 2004). In many countries, women's rights to property are attained primarily through marriage. If a marriage ends, then women are often left without any rights to land. For example, a recent study in Namibia found that 44 per cent of widows lost rights to their cattle and 41 per cent lost farm equipment after their husband's death (FAO 1996).

Many countries do not recognize that a husband can rape his wife. Marital rape stems from assumptions that women cannot refuse sex with their husband because they have given up their right to make decisions about their sexuality upon entering marriage. Researchers estimate that 25 per cent of all rapes occur within marriage (Randall and Haskings 1995). A study in India found that 34 per cent of married women reported that they had been forced to have sex with their husbands and in Zimbabwe 26 per cent of ever married women reported that they had been forced to have sex (WHO 2000). In the USA, where marital rape is considered a crime in all 50 states, many states continue to treat marital rape differently, making rape by a husband less punishable than stranger rape (Bergen 1996). Marital rape laws affect the lives of young women and also the children in the families where marital rape is occurring.

Throughout the world, young women do not receive the same rights to educational opportunities as men. Education enables women to have the same opportunities as men and to be full participants in the economy. Research demonstrates that education has a direct impact on increased labour force participation and decreased rates of fertility and children's illnesses. It is also necessary for understanding their bodies and their health, learning about contraception and learning about how sex can be fulfilling and meaningful. However, educational resources are lacking for many young women. Families may prevent young women from enrolling in schools, and governments often lack the resources or desire to intervene on behalf of young girls' right to education (USAID 2002).

Men: patriarchy and compulsory heterosexuality

The effect of patriarchy on women is well established; however, the effect of patriarchy on men is less clear but equally important to understand. Patriarchy is a system of power that is grounded in the *relationship* between men and women. Young men, therefore, learn gender roles that are compatible with women's gender roles and that place both young men and young women at risk.

To understand how men are affected by patriarchy it may be useful to utilize the notion of 'compulsory heterosexuality'. This term was first used by Rich (1980) to highlight the existence of lesbians and to understand their erasure from history and society. She argued that heterosexuality is a requisite for patriarchy to function as a system of male power. The institution of heterosexuality is comprised of unwritten but clearly codified and compulsory conventions by which men and women join in romantic relationships. Patriarchy thus assumes that all men engage in heterosexual relationships and results in women's acceptance of passive roles (Rich 1980).

In later work, Tolman (2003) extended Rich's concept of compulsory heterosexuality to young men. Her research suggests that young men encounter discourses and pressures to behave as acceptable heterosexual males that are comparable with and complementary to the discourses and pressures encountered by young women. She found that homophobia (the fear of being labelled homosexual) lay at the heart of young men's narratives about why they needed to act in coercive ways to young girls. There is a constant pressure to deflect evidence of homosexuality and to display signs of conventional masculinity as central tenets of compulsory heterosexuality as it applies to men (Connell 1995; Dowsett 1998; Kimmel and Mahler 2003; Tolman, *et al.* 2003a; Tolman *et al.* 2003b). The constant need to prove heterosexuality, for both young men and women, often makes it difficult to have healthy and equal relationships.

Compulsory heterosexuality also greatly affects the lives of young men and women attracted to the same sex. The constant push for men to prove their masculinity by engaging in sex with women, and likewise for women to prove their femininity by having a boyfriend can be detrimental. Many are unable to discuss their feelings with their parents or risk rejection when they do (Savin-Williams 1998). Feigning sexual feelings towards the opposite sex or denying one's own sexual feelings could lead many gay and lesbian young people to deny their authentic feelings in order to be accepted by others. This way of 'coping' with fears of violence and isolation that are often well founded is evident in the high suicide and depression rates that are seen among gay and lesbian young people in the USA (Rosenberg 2003). Additionally, in many countries there exists the very real threat of violence, stigma, discrimination and legal sanctions for having same-sex sexual relationships. This social rejection of attraction to the same sex may, in fact, lead to a dual life in some developing world contexts, where wives/female partners are placed at risk of HIV, by their male partner who secretly has unprotected sex with a male partner.

Working with/in gender

As we have seen, dominant gender relations seriously limit young people's opportunities. However, it is important to keep in mind that the dynamic concept of doing gender offers a reminder that gender, while deeply embedded within our society and often within ourselves, can also be malleable and challenged. Individuals and groups can and do resist the marginalizing interplay between gender and other social structures. In the following section, three case studies are offered in which individuals have taken action to reduce the effects of gender in creating health-related vulnerabilities. These case studies provide insight into possible solutions to overcome the ways that gender shapes and contributes to health-related vulnerabilities, exemplifying how individuals and groups can and do negotiate structural gender barriers through awareness and political resistance to marginalization through personal and collective action.

Girls Power Initiative, Nigeria

The Girls Power Initiative (GPI)[2] in Nigeria is an internationally renowned, non-governmental organization founded by Bene E. Madunagu and Grace Osakue in 1993. Based on their experiences as adolescent girls and as activists, they sought to empower young women, aged 10 to 18, to break free of restrictive gender roles and to arm them with information about sexuality. GPI uses a unique approach by teaching girls and encouraging open discussion about sexuality, gender roles, community action and women's rights as well as developing young women's leadership and self-reliance skills. Of particular importance is GPI's fundamental belief that educating girls to resist gender stereotypes and become active, outspoken, and 'interruptive' members of their communities is a critical part of what enables them to be sexually healthy. GPI advocacy has been instrumental in creating dialogue about sexual and reproductive health and rights among parents, educators, and policy makers in Nigeria.

GPI operates two centres, one in the southern port city of Calabar and another in Benin City and runs activity programmes in 28 schools across four states. On Sundays, both centres overflow with girls who come to socialize and build self-esteem and solidarity as they tackle issues of sexual and reproductive health and rights. More than 1,500 young women are GPI members, and a quarterly newsletter, *Girl Power*, reaches thousands more. GPI also accesses the general public with educational events and materials, including pamphlets, books and videos. The cornerstone of GPI is a

---

2 For more information on the Girls Power Initiative, go to http://www.electroniccommunity. org/GirlsPower

carefully crafted curriculum that spans several years and provides a wealth of factual information about sexuality and about reproductive health and development.

In describing her approach, Madunagu says:

> There's a social construction of who a 'good girl' is. A good girl is expected to be invisible. She's not expected to be different. In GPI, we try to help girls think critically, to question, and to realize that it is possible to be different and still be a good girl. We help the girls see beyond what they are told. For us, the issue of gender is at the bottom of everything. It is what is being used to hold the girls back. Since we think it is time the girls are no longer held back, we believe the girls should have information. They are human beings who can think, they are human beings with rights, they are human beings with responsibilities. So we approach every issue from a gender perspective.
>
> (Tolman 2003)

As a result, GPI has five objectives for the girls in their programme: to assist girls to achieve personal empowerment by rejecting gender inequality; to educate girls to take action to overcome the risks to their health arising from gender violence and discrimination; to build their leadership skills to overcome subservient roles and take on active engagement on an equal basis with their male counterparts; to sensitize girls to take social actions and educate their peers on risky behaviours harmful to their health; and to give information to assist them to overcome harmful traditions.

Women, Risk and AIDS Project, United Kingdom

The Women, Risk and AIDS Project (WRAP) was created in the 1980s by a collective of feminist sociologists in the United Kingdom. Their strategy of resistance was to produce different forms of knowledge about gender and health that could offer policy makers empirical evidence of how gender created sexual health vulnerabilities and to change public discourse about gender and sexuality. They conducted interviews with a diverse group of young women from Manchester and London regarding their sexual encounters and relationships, paying close attention to the power relations between men and women (Holland *et al.* 1990). WRAP began working in the early days of concern over HIV/AIDS. Until this time, everyday heterosexual sexual practice had mostly escaped the attention of social research. These researchers questioned the 'naturalness' of heterosexual practices and their studies sought to investigate the power relations and contradictions of normative heterosexual culture (Holland *et al.* 2000).

Their findings revealed dramatically how dominant cultural conceptions of female sexuality as passive, as devoid of desire and as subordinate to male needs and desires make it difficult for women to prevent unwanted pregnancy or negotiate safe sex (Holland *et al.* 1992). They contrast these findings with public health campaigns of the time that called for girls and women to ask their partners to wear a condom without recognizing the social repercussions of being labelled a 'slag' (slut) or potential male violence, illuminating how failing to attend to the realities of gender relations renders such efforts ineffective at best and even potentially dangerous for young women. They also reported how young women describe managing embodied sexuality in the face of a discourse of 'normal' female sexuality as disembodied that is central in reproducing gender relations. They noted that this 'possibility of disruption can offer some space for women's resistance to men's sexual power' (Holland *et al.* 1994: 23). In the later years of the project, work was extended to include young men. Research identified how norms of masculinity create pressures for young men and women in relationships, thereby increasing health-related vulnerabilities (Holland *et al.* 1998).

Working it Out, USA

By 1995, it had become clear that gay and lesbian young people in the USA were experiencing severe discrimination both at school and in their homes. The discrimination often led to alienation from friends, family and self – sometimes leading to suicide. To help young gays and lesbians accept their sexuality and to help the parents and friends of young gays and lesbians, Joyce Hunter, Director of the Community Liaison Program at the HIV Center for Clinical and Behavioral Studies in Manhattan, together with Sandra Elkin from the Media Group, Inc., set out to create a video. The video, called *Working it Out*, consisted of 14 brief scenes, for example, between a parent and their gay child, between a gay friend and a straight friend, between an older man and a younger man.

Creating the video was a highly interactive process between Hunter, six New York City organizations serving young lesbians and gay men, and young gays and lesbians themselves. This process ensured that the issues discussed in the video would be relevant and worthwhile for promoting understanding of gays' and lesbians' sexuality and acceptance of themselves and by society.

Those attending a *Working it Out* help group first watch a video scene. The discussion that follows helps build the critical thinking skills of the participants. Some typical questions for the group include: 'What were the feelings of the people in the video segment?' Participants are encouraged to share their own feelings about the scene. After discussion, a series of group exercises are conducted based on some of the themes raised by the video. For example, in one scene a presumably straight man approaches two young women and demands to know why one of the women does not want to date him. He says, 'Every time I see you, you're with her!' As he pushes his pelvis towards the girls' faces, he says 'You need a real man to show you what it's like'. Following this scene participants are asked to write (but not necessarily to send) letters to those who have harassed them.

Working it Out has made its way from New York City to Utah where the Gay and Lesbian Community Center draws clients from across northern Utah, as well as parts of Idaho, Colorado and Nevada. *Working it Out* began there in 2000 and has continued with great success, though so far only with participants aged over 18. Parental consent is required for minors, and in Utah, a US state in which the majority of the population is Mormon, a religion that bans homosexuality, parental consent for this kind of activity is hard to come by (Pratt 2002).

Together the three case studies illustrate innovative techniques that actively engage individuals to think about and to change the gender options they have been given in their communities. Through gaining knowledge and understanding of gender relationships, individuals feel compelled to seek gender equality. Additionally, young women and men learn how gender shapes their lives and learn how to take steps to protect themselves from some of the detrimental health effects that gender produces.

Conclusions

In this chapter, we have introduced the basic concepts of gender and patriarchy and illustrated how both can lead to detrimental sexual health vulnerabilities for young people. Gender 'functions' in different ways in different parts of the world; however, its effect is often very similar – to diminish sexual health. Both complying with and going against gender norms can make young people vulnerable. However, innovative approaches to gender with young people have not only enlightened young women and young men to how gender works in their lives, but have also used gender as a means to enact change and to improve health in the lives of young people.

References

AAUW (1993) *Hostile hallways: The AAUW (American Association of University Women) survey on sexual harassment in America's schools*, Washington, DC: AAUW Educational Foundation Research.

Allen, S.M. (1982) 'Adolescent Pregnancy among 11–15 year-old Girls in the Parish of Manchester'. Unpublished Ph.D. dissertation. Kingston: University of the West Indies. Cited in MacCormack, C.P. and A. Draper 'Social and cognitive aspects of female sexuality in Jamaica', in P. Caplan (ed.) *The Cultural Construction of Sexuality*, London: Tavistock Publications.

Amaro, H. (1995) 'Love, sex, and power: Considering women's realities in HIV prevention', *American Psychologist*, 50(6): 437–47.

Beadnell, B., Baker, S.A., Morrison, D.M. and Knox, K. (2000) 'HIV/STD risk factors for women with violent male partners', *Sex Roles,* 42: 661–89.

Bergen, R.K. (1996) *Wife rape: Understanding the response of survivors and service providers*, Thousand Oaks, CA: Sage.

Bianchi, S.M. (1999) 'Feminization and juvenilization of poverty: Trends, relative risks, causes, and consequences', *Annual Review of Sociology*, 25: 307–44.

Browne, A. (1993) 'Violence against women by male partners: Prevalence, outcomes, and policy implications', *American Psychologist*, 48: 1077–87.

Buss, D.M. (1999) 'Sexual conflict: Evolutionary insights into feminism and the "battle of the sexes"', in D.M. Buss and N.M. Malamuth (eds) *Sex, power, conflict: Evolutionary and feminist perspectives*, New York: Oxford University Press, pp. 296–318.

Butler, J. (1993) *Bodies that matter: On the discursive limits of sex*, New York: Routledge.

Carballo, M. and Simic, S. (1996) 'Health in countries torn by conflict: Lessons from Sarajevo', *Lancet,* 348: 872–5.

Cohen, M., Deamant, C., Barkan, S., Richardson, J., Young, M., Holman, S., Anastos, K., Cohen, J. and Melnick, S. (2000) 'Domestic violence and childhood sexual abuse in HIV-infected women and women at risk for HIV', *American Journal of Public Health,* 90: 560–5.

Connell, R.W. (1995) *Masculinities*, Berkeley: University of California Press.

Connell, R.W. (1999) 'Making gendered people: Bodies, identities, sexualities', in

M.M. Ferree, J. Lorder and B.B. Hess (eds) *Revisioning Gender*, Thousand Oaks, CA: Sage, pp. 449–72.

Dickson, N., Paul, C., Herbison, P. and Silva, P. (1998) 'First sexual intercourse: Age, coercion, and later regrets reported by a birth cohort', *British Medical Journal*, 316: 29–33.

Dowsett, G.W. (1998) 'Wusses and willies: masculinity and contemporary sexual politics', *Journal of Interdisciplinary Gender Studies*, 3: 9–22.

England, P. and Farkas, G. (1986) *Households, employment and gender: A social, economic and demographic view*, New York: Aldine.

FAO (1996) *Namibia: Women, Agriculture and Rural Development* (http://www.fao.org/sd/WPdirect/WPan0002.html).

Gough, K. (1975) 'The origin of the family', in R.R. Reiter (ed.) *Toward an anthropology of women*, New York: Monthly Review Press.

Gurungr, G. (1998) 'Nepalis start to "make a noise" about sex trafficking. Online at (http://www.mahilaweb.org.np/trafficking/report_summary/trafficking-panos.htm).

Heise, L. and Elias, C. (1995) 'Transforming AIDS prevention to meet women's needs: A focus on developing countries', *Social Science Medicine*, 40: 931–43.

Holland, J., Ramazanoglu, C., Scott, S. and Thomson, R. (1990) 'Sex, gender and power: Young women's sexuality in the shadow of AIDS', *Sociology of Health Illness*, 12: 336–50.

Holland, J., Ramazanoglu, C., Scott, S., Sharpe, S. and Thomson, R. (1992) 'Risk, power and the possibility of pleasure: Young women and safer sex', *AIDS Care*, 4: 273–83.

Holland, J., Ramazanoglu, C., Scott, S., Sharpe, S. and Thomson, R. (1994) 'Sex, gender and power: Young women's sexuality in the shadow of AIDS', in B. Rauh (ed.) *AIDS: Readings on a global crisis*, London: Allyn and Bacon, pp. 336–50.

Holland, J., Ramazanoglu, C., Sharpe, S. and Thomson, R. (1998) *The Male in the Head*, London: Tufnell Press.

Holland, J., Ramazanoglu, C., Sharpe, S. and Thomson, R. (2000) 'Deconstructing virginity – young people's accounts of first sex', *Sexual and Relationship Therapy*, 15: 221–32.

HRW (Human Rights Watch) (2001) *Hatred in the hallways: Violence and discrimination against lesbian, gay, bisexual, and transgender students in U.S. schools*, New York: Human Rights Watch.

Kalichman, S.C., Williams, E.A., Cherry, C., Belcher, L. and Nachimson, D. (1998) 'Sexual coercion, domestic violence, negotiating condom use among low-income African American Women', *Journal of Women's Health*, 7: 371–8.

Kimmel, M.S. and Mahler, M. (2003) 'Adolescent masculinity, homophobia, and violence: Random school shootings, 1982–2001', *American Behavioral Scientist*, 46: 1439–58.

Lee, V.E., Croninger, R.G., Linn, E. and Chen, X. (1996) 'The culture of sexual harassment in secondary schools', *American Education Research Journal*, 32: 383–417.

Mane, P. and Aggleton, P. (2001) 'Gender and HIV/AIDS: What do men have to do with it?' *Current Sociology*, 49: 23–37.

Pearson, R. (1994) *Gender relations, capitalism and Third World industrialization in capitalism and development*, London: Routledge.

Pearson, R. (1998) '"Nimble fingers" revisited: Reflections on women and Third World industrialization in the late twentieth century', in C. Jackson and R. Pearson (eds) *Feminist visions of development: Gender analysis and policy*, London: Routledge, pp. 171–88.

Pleck, J.H. (1987) 'The theory of male sex-role identity: Its rise and fall, 1936 to the present', in H. Brod (ed.) *The making of masculinities: The new men's studies*, Boston: Allen Unwin, pp. 21–38.

Pratt, D. (2002) 'Working it Out: Scenes from the lives of gay and lesbian youth', *Body Positive, XV*, New York: Body Positive Publications.

Randall, M. and Haskings, L. (1995) 'Sexual violence in women's lives', *Violence Against Women*, 1: 6–31.

Rao Gupta, G. (2000) *Gender, sexuality, and HIV/AIDS: The what, the why, and the how*, Washington, DC: International Center for Research on Women.

Rich, A. (1980) 'Compulsory heterosexuality and lesbian existence', *Signs: Journal of Women in Culture and Society*, 5: 631–60.

Rich, A. (1999) 'Compulsory heterosexuality and lesbian existence', in R. Parker and P. Aggleton (eds) *Culture, society and sexuality: A reader*, London: UCL Press, pp. 199–225.

Rosenberg, M. (2003) 'Recognizing gay, lesbian, and transgender teens in a child and adolescent psychiatry practice', *Journal of the American Academy of Child and Adolescent Psychiatry*, 42: 1517–21.

Savin-Williams, R.C. (1998) 'Lesbian, gay and bisexual youths' relationships with their parents', in C. Patterson and A.R. D'Augelli (eds) *Lesbian, gay and bisexual identities in families*, New York: Oxford University Press, pp. 75–98.

Scott, J.W. (1999) 'Gender as a useful category of historical analysis', in R. Parker and P. Aggleton (eds) *Culture, society and sexuality: A reader*, London: UCL Press, pp. 57–75.

Spence, J.T. (1993) 'Gender-related traits and gender ideology: Evidence for multifactorial theory', *Journal of Personality and Social Psychology*, 64: 624–35.

Stein, N. (1999) *Classrooms and courtrooms: Facing sexual harassment in K-12 schools*, New York: Teacher's College Press.

Thomson, R. and Holland, J. (1994) 'Younger women and safer (hetero)sex: Context, constraints and strategies', in C. Kitzinger and S. Wilkinson (eds) *Women and health: Feminist perspectives*, London: Falmer, pp. 13–32.

Tjaden, P. and Thoennes, N. (2000) *Full report of the prevalence, incidence, and consequences of violence against women*, Washington, DC: National Center of Justice.

Tolman, D.L. (2003) 'Empowering girls: Nigerian activists focus on gender and sexuality', *Wellsley Centers for Women: Research and Action Report, Summer/ Spring* (http://www.wcwonline.org/o-rr24-2c.html).

Tolman, D.L., Spencer, R., Rosen-Reynoso, M., and Porche, M.V. (2003a) 'Sowing the seeds of violence in heterosexual relationships: Early adolescents narrate compulsory heterosexuality', *Journal of Social Issues*, 59: 159–79.

Tolman, D.L., Striepe, M.I. and Harmon, T. (2003b) 'Gender matters: Constructing a model of adolescent sexual health', *Journal of Sex Research*, 40: 4–12.

UNAIDS (1999) *Gender and HIV/AIDS: Taking stock of research programmes*, Geneva: UNAIDS.

UNAIDS (2003) *Men and boys can make a difference in the response to the HIV/AIDS epidemic*, Brasilia, Brazil: United Nations.

UNAIDS (2004) 'Aids epidemic update 2004' (http://www.unaids.org/wad2004/report.html).

Upton, R.L. (2003) '"Women Have No Tribe": Connecting carework, gender, and migration in an era of HIV/AIDS in Botswana', *Gender and Society*, 17: 314–22.

USAID (2002) *USAID (United States Agency for International Development) Girls' education initiatives in Guatemala, Guinea, Mali, Morocco and Peru: A performance review*, Arlington, Virginia: USAID.

West, C. and Fenstermaker, S. (1995) 'Doing difference', *Gender and Society*, 9: 8–37.

West, C. and Zimmerman, D.H. (1987) 'Doing gender', *Gender and Society*, 1: 125–51.

WHO (2000) *Violence against women and HIV/AIDS: Setting the research agenda*, Geneva: World Health Organization.

Wingood, G.M. and DiClemente, R.J. (1997) 'The effects of an abusive primary partner on the condom use and sexual negotiation practices of African-American women', *American Journal of Public Health*, 87: 1016–18.

Chapter 4

Ethnicity, culture, drugs and sex

Carol Jenkins

Race, culture and ethnicity are central to understanding young people's use of both licit and illicit drugs. They also link closely to popular perceptions of the use of drugs among young people, including the interaction between drugs and sex. This chapter discusses a range of relevant issues so as to distinguish more clearly between fact and fiction, and so as to lay the ground for more appropriate future responses. It begins with some discussion of what each of these terms means and how they are used.

Concepts of race, ethnicity and culture are complex. Culture is a broad concept referring to learned ways of being in a society of people, including ideas, actions and artifacts. Contrary to what many believe, race is a cultural construct, used very differently in different parts of the world.[1] Race, when referring to humans, is essentially a modern concept used primarily to legitimate social inequalities. Biologically, it has no sound meaning with regard to humans because the human species has not been divided into isolated groups for long enough to evolve into sub-species or races. Ethnicity, particularly in western societies, is increasingly a formal politico-demographic marker, often used to make a statement about one's sense of self in relation to a larger society. This is particularly true where self-identification prevails, as in the case of UK, Australian and US censuses. In some rural societies, for example small groups of people living along a mountain range in Papua New Guinea, ethnic identity can be fluid and a person may use one identity in certain situations and another in other situations.

Ethnicity is also a fuzzy concept that overlaps at times with concepts of race, minority, nationality and tribe. While it may have some importance to the individual, it is often misused in data collection and analysis – particularly in studies that attempt to assess the prevalence of behaviours such as substance use among different groups of young people. Indeed, much

---

1 Genetic diversity in drug-metabolizing enzymes does exist, affecting the way a drug, such as codeine or alcohol, is experienced, and these are sometimes distributed along ethnic lines; but dietary and other environmental factors also interact (Lin and Poland 2000).

public discourse concerning young people, sex and drugs is tinged with subtle racism and scapegoating. This has been especially true in the USA and has had enormous influence on drug policy through the years. Within such discourses, terms such as Asian, Black, Hispanic, White Non-Hispanic, Native American, and so on are often used with scant regard to the diversity of practice and experience subsumed within each of these categories, and often with little regard to the truth. Among school aged young people, at least, surveys consistently show the greater use of any illicit drug by US white students than African-American or Hispanic students (Johnston *et al.* 2003b).

A clear example of the extent of misrepresentation of drug use is provided by the analysis of how a fabricated story of a young African-American heroin addict could be so easily believed.

In the *Washington Post*, in 1980, a story appeared about Jimmy, an 8-year-old African-American heroin addict. It created an enormous stir and almost won the author a Pulitzer Prize but turned out to be a hoax. 'When seen as part of the historical pattern of news coverage of drug issues, the Pulitzer Prize-winning fraud was less a lapse than part of a long tradition. Throughout the twentieth century the media helped foment a series of drug scares, each magnifying drug menaces well beyond their objective dimensions. From the turn of the century into the 1920s, the yellow journalism of the Hearst newspapers, for example, offered a steady stream of ruin and redemption melodramas. These depicted one or another chemical villain, typically in the hands of a 'dangerous class' or racial minority, as responsible for the end of Western civilization. In the 1930s, newspapers repeated unsubstantiated claims that marijuana, 'the killer weed', led users, Mexicans in particular, to violence. . . . In the 1960s, the press somehow re-made 'killer weed' into 'the drop-out drug', and spread other misleading reports that LSD broke chromosomes and yielded two-headed babies. In the 1970s, the press again falsely reported that 'angel dust' or PCP gave users such superhuman strength that the police needed new stun guns to subdue them. In 1986, the press and politicians once again joined forces on crack cocaine use among the black underclass. The drug was unknown outside of a few neighborhoods in a few cities until newspapers, magazines, and TV networks blanketed the nation with horror stories that described the crack high. In each of these drug scares, the media has consistently erred on the side of the sensational and dutifully repeated the self-serving scare stories of politicians in search of safe issues on which to take strong stands.

> The media that might have served as a source of credible warnings about the risks of drug abuse were dismissed with derision by the very users they needed to reach.
>
> (Adapted from Reinarman and Duskin 1992)

The real-world biocultural complexity of people and their various identities cannot be captured in tick-off boxes of questionnaire forms. As a factor that could be used to explain a particular social or behavioral trait, terms like Hispanic or Latino in the Americas are next to useless, because they include every Spanish-speaking people from Mexico through the Caribbean to the tip of South America. The cultural differences between a Mexican of Mayan descent and a Cuban of African descent are vast, and totally lost in the official terminology of ethnic identity. Similarly, in the UK, the term white can encompass recent migrants, such as Portuguese and Italians, living in close-knit ethnic communities and simply unseen in the usual ethnicity matrix (Kalunta-Crumpton 2003).

In much research on drugs and sex among youth, ethnic labels are often confounded with other factors, such as poverty, discrimination and institutional racism, crowding, low levels of education, migration status, political subordination and so on. As a result, findings regarding etiology, patterns of substance use and its effects often explain very little. Cultural processes, on the other hand, while harder to define and to describe, may have greater salience in explaining global patterns of drug use and sexual activity among young people. The discussion that follows will examine the interaction of ethnicity, as usually defined, and selected cultural processes as they apply to drug use and the interaction of drugs and sex among young people in different parts of the world today.

Culture and psychotropic drugs: transcendence and getting high

The use of mind-altering drugs has an ancient history. Societies around the world have found that certain plants or other substances affect the mind in ways that are valued for their capacity to transform perceptions, moods or emotions. Perhaps as a result, traditional patterns of use, often sacred and managed through ritual, have been institutionalized and not perceived as social or health problems.

Globally, mind-altering substances have been used in a wide variety of rituals, including induction as a sorcerer, initiations into healing cults, by shamans in healing or preventive rites, and so on. Many have been used in rituals marking the entry to adulthood, or were permitted to those who had grown out of adolescence (Grob and Dobkin de Rios 1992). This traditional pharmacopia included opium, coca, numerous hallucinogens and stimulants, as well as various alcoholic drinks.

Some religious and healing rituals also continue to use mind-altering drugs in traditional frameworks, but the world is more secular than earlier. There is now a large number of societies in which substance use is maintained as a social as opposed to a religious institution, is seen as relatively non-problematic, and is gradually taught to young people (usually males only) under managed conditions – for example, *kava* drinking in Melanesia or *qat* chewing in the Arabian Peninsula and the Horn of Africa. In many societies, the social drinking of alcohol, even binge drinking, is a rite of passage for young men, with young women following close behind. The well-known widespread ideology and practice of Rastafarianism and its association with marijuana crosses over boundaries of religion, identity politics, and popular music.

The number of mind-altering drugs has vastly increased over the centuries and become far more accessible to the general population. Under these circumstances, for many people, the desire to transcend the here-and-now is less a religious motive than a wish to escape any of a number of states, for example, destitution, abusive relationships, pain, boredom, material deprivation, subordination, depression, loneliness, ill-health, hunger, low self-esteem, the perceived lack of love and so on. But, for the majority of young people in many societies, trying out different psychoactive substances is clearly more of a social activity than anything else and may not be associated with low self-esteem, deviance or criminality. From binge drinking to ecstasy raves, drug use during holidays, at weekends and in school breaks is commonplace, considered normal by many adults and even institutionalized (Apostolopoulos *et al.* 2002, Bellis *et al.* 2004). Increasingly, in many societies, young people are trying out drugs at earlier ages and using them longer. During the course of these drug-using careers, a few may become seriously dependent, while others negotiate a lifestyle that allows 'soma' holidays amidst hard work, intense schooling, and eventually even a family life and active career (Cohen and Sas 1994, Parker 2003). After many years of managed use, these people may be labeled functional drug users, though functionality is hard to predict in the young user.

Health consequences, such as transient side-effects and longer-term changes in the brain and body, including dependency, may adhere to the continuing use of many such substances. Each substance has its own set of chemical effects and individuals may respond quite differently to different drugs and different doses. However, the setting in which drug use occurs – including aspects of the local culture, the health and nutritional status of the population, the physical environment, social networks, venues of use, access to health care, the legal status of a drug, local law enforcement procedures, and the longer-term opportunity structures in a community – has a considerable influence on the likelihood of negative outcomes. Frequency of use may be driven by these externalities.

One of the major forces causing negative outcomes is the intensified criminalization of substance use. Over the last century, political and economic forces have driven an increasing repression of the use of psychotropic drugs among young people globally. There is often little relationship between the nature of a drug and its effects to the degree of prohibition. More often, political and economic forces determine which drugs people have access to, than do concerns about health or well-being. This is as true today as it was in the past, when coffee was outlawed by Prussia's King Frederick to bolster sagging beer prices.

While there is a serious scientific effort to sort out exactly what different drugs do to the human mind and body, official drug policies do not ordinarily base their premises on science. Logic and evidence notwithstanding, nicotine, the most addictive substance known, remains legal throughout the world, while drugs with little documented harm or addictive potential, such as marijuana, are widely prohibited. This has created a serious gap in the credibility of drug education efforts, especially in the USA. Consequently, few have shown any success at all in reducing demand (Botvin *et al.* 1996, Kreft and Brown 1998).

In 1998, the UN General Assembly Special Session on Drugs committed itself to a drug-free world by 2008, but illicit drug use continues to grow and change shape despite an intensive investment in the 'war on drugs' (Jelsma 2003). Importantly, the war on drugs approach, supporting an increasing army of crop eradicators and drug police, has done little to reduce heroin or cocaine availability in the USA to the present day (Kane 2001).

The effects of these policies on each new generation of young people are profound. Policy makers generally continue to respond with punitive measures and 'Just say No'-type educational messages in complete denial of their inefficacy. In the USA, there is some evidence that intense scare tactics concerning ecstasy, a popular club drug among youth, may have reduced usage levels after the year 2000 (Johnston *et al.* 2004). In Thailand, violent anti-drug campaigns have recently reduced, but not eliminated, the supply of amphetamine-type substances (Rojanaphruk 2004). But new drugs are discovered periodically and old ones gain renewed popularity (e.g. methamphetamine in the early 2000s), without the provision of realistic population-directed drug education.

Overall, the use of illicit drugs by young people has not diminished and, in some regions, for example in Russia and the countries of the Commonwealth of Independent States, it is definitely on the increase. The threats and benefits associated with 'getting high' have not been managed well by society's policy makers, leaving an enormous gap to be filled by other cultural processes.

A Maldivian Tale

After a focus group discussion ended about youth, sex and drugs with a group of young men between 16 and 22 years of age on a small island in the Maldives, one young man wanted to speak privately. He started, with his head down, to say that he was in love with a girl who was 'chasing' heroin, as were many young people on the island. He did not use heroin and nearly cried as he asked how he could manage to resist his girlfriend's influence. She criticized him for listening to the wrong music, for wearing the wrong type of trousers, and so on. He just wasn't one of her group and didn't fit, yet he loved her, he said, and was very distraught. His distress belied the great need of many young people to be able to speak of these issues with a non-judgmental adult. There were no such services anywhere in the country, despite very high reported rates of heroin use among the young people of the Maldives.

Processes of social exclusion and inclusion

The desire to be connected to others or included in any of a variety of social arrangements seems rooted in human nature, but the many ways in which young people bond or form groups emerge from contemporary sociocultural processes. Numerous studies show how a sense of social exclusion and the desire for inclusion influence both drug use and sexual behaviours, far more than ethnic identity. Recent studies of young people in school in the USA consistently show higher illicit drug use rates among white youth than among African-Americans or Hispanics, indicating that minority ethnic status per se is not a determinant of illicit drug use (Johnston *et al.* 2003b).[2] Studies of school drop-outs in both the UK (Jeffrey *et al.* 2001) and the USA (Swaim *et al.* 1997) show higher illicit drug use rates than among young people in school, especially among minority youth. Among homeless young people, those without social support networks were found to have significantly greater likelihood of using illicit drugs and practicing transactional or 'survival' sex with multiple partners than those having social networks (Ennett *et al.* 1999).

Young people in most countries have to learn to manage sex and drugs safely with little constructive support from the adults in their own cultural

2 In the USA, Native American youth have higher levels of marijuana use than all other groups, but survey results are not strictly comparable to the repeated national Monitoring the Future surveys of other high school students. Also, out of 550 officially recognized tribes, there are no drug use data on over 200 tribes.

environments. According to social learning theory, young people who have role models and receive social approval for deviant behaviors, are more likely to adopt them (Bandura 1977). Hence, social researchers have placed great emphasis on the often-demonstrated strength of peer pressure as a mechanism that pushes young people into risky behaviors.

Less often acknowledged is the way in which authorized cultural practices also play a role in establishing models for behavior. The widespread use of licit drugs to manage levels of psychic energy, moods and stress in western societies creates a high background load of psychotropic drug-use role models. An analysis in the USA of government-subsidized (Medicaid) and health maintenance organization prescribing practices for young people between 1987 and 1996 showed that psychotropic medication prevalence for young people increased two to three fold, nearly to adult levels, and included mood stabilizers, anticonvulsants, alpha-agonists, neuroleptics, antidepressants, hypnotics, and stimulants (Zito et al. 2003). Another study found children were more likely to receive psychotropic drugs if their parents took them (Hong and Shepherd 1996).

In many societies, young people form sub-cultures that ritualize illicit drug use as part of a larger identity process. Through participation in these sub-cultures, young people have a chance to try out drugs and sex as well as a variety of belief systems in a peer-managed setting. Globally, youth sub-cultures have evolved, at least in part, as a form of resistance to authoritarian and repressive social forces, or, in certain settings, in response to marked intergenerational conflict. Music styles and types of musical events play a large role in the social organization of these sub-cultures. Specific drugs of choice have become associated with some of these youth sub-cultures, although, in most cases, alcohol and marijuana predominate. Researchers point out the importance of different music styles to identity formation among young people and the accompanying dress style, body decorations and use of substances at music events (Aquatius, Boitel and Grenouillet 2002).

These have proliferated in western societies, and, through globalized communications, are spreading widely. Some are associated with specific ethnic groups, but by no means all. Raves are associated with the use of ecstasy (MDMA), LSD and other psychedelics and stimulants. Raves began in the UK and have spread throughout much of Europe, North America and elsewhere. Ravers tend to eschew alcohol, drinking water instead (Birgit and Krüger n.d., Seppälä and Salasuo n.d., Gilman 1994). The heavy metal crowd use ecstasy, marijuana and methamphetamine, listen to heavy metal rock, and increasingly have their own venues in numerous countries. 'Gangsta rap' music defines a sub-culture with a jargon, a dress style and, in the USA, is associated with the use of crack cocaine and African-Americans (Rose 1994, Krohn and Suazo 1995).

In some poorer countries, home-grown (or maybe colonized) youth sub-cultures have developed that seem more or less equivalent to their western counterparts, for example, *roqueros* and *kakos* (also known as *raperos*) in Puerto Rico (Rivera 2002). Ethnicity plays a role in the dissemination of these sub-cultures in that the exported image of rapper African-Americans appeals to Africans more than do images of white Americans and Europeans. As one Namibian youngster replied when asked about what influenced him, 'Movies from America influence me. I want to be a nigger from America and dress like Tupac and talk like them – the gangsters' (Soul Beat Africa 2003).

Class and ethnicity are factors that help define youth sub-cultures. Clothes, music, language and other markers help define social status in all of these sub-cultures. In many settings, drugs also mean earning money (Sherman and Latkin 2002). Drugs cost money and poor young people cannot afford the more expensive designer drugs that the middle and upper classes can. Among Central Asian youth, drugs have become a part of the lifestyle and connote the image of power, being cool and having money. One young Tajik made a statement that could have been made by many young people around the world:

> We grew up seeing the drug mafia openly dealing, the big cars and tough guys, just like the movies. In schools and universities students went to classes with guns and threatened any teacher not giving them the best marks. People were injecting drugs publicly. Now it is all hidden. Just two or three big guys control the whole thing, pay off the police and business continues but in a hidden way. But everybody knows a lot of people made their fortune in the drug business and it continues.
>
> (International Crisis Group 2003: 28)

More recently, the continued commonplace use of illicit recreational or club drugs among young people, especially in Western Europe, Australia, Canada and the USA, has led some observers to point out that the practice now cannot be associated so closely with delinquent or deviant behavior (Duff 2003, Parker *et al.* 1998). Indeed, a little less than half of all twelfth graders in the USA report having tried an illicit substance and this proportion has barely changed in almost a decade (Johnston *et al.* 2004). The popularity of different drugs does shift, however, and the perceived risks and benefits are quite specific to particular drugs. While these substances may be illegal, many young people who are well adjusted and achieving individuals perceive no problem in the recreational controlled use of one or more of these drugs, such as marijuana, tranquilizers or amphetamine. The normalization of drug use, or at least drug experimenting, in youth cultures and lifestyles has widespread currency, particularly among young people themselves.

Ethnicity and negative consequences

In complex societies, being a member of a subordinate ethnic or sex/gender group that is socially excluded and marginalized is often associated with increased negative consequences of drug use. Ethnicity per se, however, may not be the defining factor marking societal exclusion. Among homeless young people, sexual minorities such as gay, lesbian, bisexual and transgender young people report leaving home more frequently, being victimized more often, using highly addictive substances more frequently, having higher rates of psychopathology, and having more sexual partners than their heterosexual peers (Cochran *et al.* 2002). Such young people are more marginalized than others and may seek inclusion and acceptance, to some degree, through the use of illicit drugs in self-defined groups.

In the USA, and despite the fact that a higher proportion of whites report the use of illicit drugs than other groups, a far greater proportion of African-Americans and Latino-Americans go to prison on drug-related charges.[3] African-Americans constitute 13 percent of all current (past month) drug users, but 35 percent of those arrested for drug possession, 55 percent of persons convicted, and 74 percent of people sent to prison. Nationally, Latinos comprise almost half of those arrested for marijuana offences and Native Americans comprise almost two-thirds of those prosecuted for criminal offences in federal courts (Human Rights Watch 2000). Similar issues underlie the extremely disproportionate rates of incarceration of indigenous Australians, with it being estimated that Aborigines are 27 times more likely to be in custody than non-Aborigines (Davis 1999) and five times more likely to acquire HIV (Casella 2002).

The devastating health consequences of the war on drugs are more dramatic in communities of color. Despite the proven success of needle/ syringe exchange and other injecting equipment distribution schemes in reducing the spread of HIV, many areas of the world still do not permit them to operate. According to the US Centers for Disease Control, African-Americans account for 37 percent of all AIDS cases and 41 percent of those cases are injection-related. Latinos account for 19.2 percent of all AIDS cases and more than 44 percent of those cases are injection-related. Yet African-Americans only comprise 12.2 percent of the population and Latinos comprise only 11.9 percent of the population. Within injecting drug user networks in New York City, the Latino of African descent suffers greater racial discrimination than other Latinos or other African-Americans, and this greater subordination is associated with higher levels of HIV infection (Friedman *et al.* 1998b).

---

3 It is not really certain that levels of reporting are equally without bias across these ethnic groups. It may be that minority persons underreport. In the USA, suggestions have been made to attempt to redress this possibility in future surveys.

In their definitive review of drug use and ethnic/racial minorities in the USA, the National Institute on Drug Abuse makes the following statement:

> Available information indicates that use of these drugs may be harming the health and social well-being of these population groups disproportionately, based on their reported use of these drugs. Adverse consequences suffered by some of our racial/ethnic minority populations include excess risks of arrest, conviction, and incarceration for drug-related crimes, against a background of statistics that suggest no excess involvement of illegal drug use. These adverse consequences extend to overrepresentation in statistics of drug-related morbidity and mortality, disruption of educational achievement (e.g. greater failure to earn the regular high-school diploma), and social disadvantage.
>
> (NIDA 2003: 139)

Seeking pleasure: sex and drugs

While all individuals seek pleasure, some cultures are more open while others more narrowly define the range of acceptable pleasures. Sexual pleasure is permitted to children in some cultures, and is considered harmless play. Adolescence barely exists as a social age-based category in many societies and the transition from child directly to adult may be marked with rituals, usually – but not always – when indicators of sexual maturation reveal change. Ethnic or cultural differences in the initiation of adult sexual practice are fairly well documented, but are not widely associated with drug use. The interaction of drug use and sex is influenced by a complex set of factors, including economic need, gender power differentials, network characteristics, local concepts of masculinity, and changing socially defined arenas of pleasure, among a myriad of other factors (Flom *et al.* 2001).

One of the chief sought-after effects of drugs is disinhibition. Users report the expectation of enhanced sexual pleasure in association with almost every type of drug, including alcohol, heroin, amphetamine, marijuana, LSD, tranquilizers or even *qat*. These expectations can function as autosuggestions and therefore work fairly well, at least at times. Most studies concerned with the interaction of drugs and sex find nonspecific associations with negative outcomes, for example, a low rate of condom use among young people who last had sex while high on drugs (usually alcohol). When studies do not control for type of drug, type of partner, setting, availability of condoms and other important factors, it remains difficult to assess the real impact of drug use per se on the practice of safer sex.

Violence and coercive sex sometimes appear to be associated with drug use but again this remains difficult to confirm as a causal factor. The practice of specific sexual acts – such as heterosexual anal intercourse and group sex – if considered unusual or stigmatized in a particular society, may be associated with disinhibiting influences, such as drugs. One study of young African-American and Latina women in New York showed a statistically significant relationship of unprotected anal intercourse and use of illicit drugs, mainly marijuana and cocaine (Friedman *et al.* 2001).

Individual drugs can have quite specific effects. Recently, concern has been expressed about the association between methamphetamine use and unsafe sex among younger gay and other homosexually active men, including those living with HIV (Degenhardt and Topp 2003). In Thailand and other parts of southeast Asia, the use of amphetamine-type substances has sharply risen over the past five years, leading many to be concerned that sexual risk-taking under the influence of 'speed' will increase and lead to many new HIV infections. In the USA, studies of young people's drug use show the same trends in all major ethnic categories, i.e. a higher proportion with multiple sexual partners and lower levels of condom use at last sex when crack or other cocaine was used before sex, compared to either marijuana or no drugs (NIDA 2003).

Overall, younger or newer drug users appear to have higher sexual transmission risks than older ones. A study in Bangladesh (Government of Bangladesh 2000) examined the sexual risks of buprenorphine (a synthetic opioid) injectors in Dhaka and separated the newer injectors (<=2 years) from the older injectors. Newer injectors were at greater risk than older ones on many counts. They were also younger (median age = 26.6 vs. 38.0), far more often single (73.8 percent vs. 7.3 percent), and far more sexually active. Many more had been to sex workers during both the previous month (73.3 percent vs. 21.2 percent) and the previous year (93.2 percent vs. 54.5 percent) at over twice the frequency (mean number of sex workers last year: 9.2 vs. 4.4). During the previous month among the newer injectors, 26 percent had participated in group sex (multiple males and a single female or male), while only 7.1 percent of older injectors had. A much larger proportion of new injectors were bisexually active as well in the past year, 21.2 percent vs. 5.0 percent, a larger proportion having had sex with men (6.8 percent vs. 1.1 percent) and with *hijras* [transgender individuals] (16.4 percent vs. 3.9 percent). Furthermore, last year 15.8 percent sold sex for cash or drugs, vs. 0.7 percent among those who had injected for a longer time. But, importantly, levels of condom use and needle sharing were significantly higher among the younger men. Similar results have been reported elsewhere (Friedman *et al.* 1998a).

Conclusions

Harm reduction for drug users, particularly injection drug users, has shown clear success in reducing rates of HIV infection. However, in many parts of the world, governments wish to enforce a 'no drugs–no sex' policy for young people. Primary risk reduction by reducing demand for drugs to zero or remaining abstinent sexually, has recently attracted increased government funding. Yet, there is little in human history to support the notion that there will ever be drug-free, or for that matter, sex-free, young populations.

Many negative social phenomena are associated with illicit drug use but causation is extremely difficult to impute. Cultural factors may indeed structure drug use, but economic and social factors seem a great deal stronger. Where young people have little hope for their future, vulnerability to drug abuse is likely to be higher than where youth have a chance for a decent life. One factor found in the most recent national survey of substance use among young people in the USA showed a significant and relatively large protective effect among all ethnic groups and for all drug use (even smoking cigarettes) of intending to go to a full four-year college (Johnston *et al.* 2003a). In most other nations, such studies have not taken place and the intention to attain a higher education may mean less than the intention of being employed, or the goal of owning land to farm, or a boat to use for earning an income.

Far greater investment in understanding local cultural processes is needed to develop effective programmes with and for the world's diverse population of young people, and especially in circumstances where the effects of poverty, social exclusion and inequality are most firmly felt. Ultimately, a better understanding is required both of normative patterns of substance use, the functionality or otherwise of specific forms of use, and the factors associated with serious harm, both for the self and for others. Disentangling the complex nexus of correlates, determinants and contextual influences on the relationship between drug use and sex-related risk and vulnerability will require time and effort. Investment in more humane, pragmatic and culturally responsive policies and programmes will, however, benefit rich and poorer countries alike.

References

Apostolopoulos, Y., Sonmez, S. and Yu, C. (2002) 'HIV-risk behaviors of American spring break vacationers: a case of situational disinhibition?' *International Journal of STDs and AIDS*, 13: 733–43.

Aquatius, S., Boitel, L. and Grenouillet, G. (2002) 'The use of psychoactive products in rock culture party environments', *Trends* No. 27, December. Online. Available HTTP: <http://www.drogues.gouv.fr/uk/professionnal/pdf/tend27.pdf> (accessed 9 January 2004).

Bandura, A. (1977) *Social Learning Theory*, Englewood Cliffs, NY: Prentice-Hall.

Bellis, M., Hughes, K., Thomson, R. and Bennett, A. (2004) 'Sexual behaviour of young people in international tourist resorts', *Sexually Transmitted Infections*, 80: 43–7.

Birgit, R. and Krüger, H. (n.d.) 'Raver's paradise? German youth cultures in the 1990's'. Online. Available HTTP: <http://www.birgitrichard.de/texte/dance.htm> (accessed 9 January 2004).

Botvin, G.J., Baker, E., Dusenbury, L. and Botvin, M. (1996) 'Long-term follow-up results of a randomized drug abuse prevention trial in a white, middle-class population', *Journal of the American Medical Association*, 273: 1106–12.

Casella, N. (2002) 'Australia: Aborigines leading in risk of HIV', *Perth Sunday Times* 07.14.02. Online. Available HTTP: <http://www.thebody.com/cdc/news_updates_archive/july18_02/aborigines_hiv.html> (accessed 3 April 2004).

Cochran, B., Stewart, A., Ginzler, J. and Cauce, A. (2002) 'Challenges faced by homeless sexual minorities: comparison of gay, lesbian, bisexual, and transgender homeless adolescents with their heterosexual counterparts', *American Journal of Public Health*, 92: 773–7.

Cohen, P. and Sas, A. (1994) 'Cocaine use in Amsterdam in non deviant subcultures', *Dependency Research*, 2: 71–94.

Davis, B. (1999) *The inappropriateness of the criminal justice system – an indigenous Australian criminological perspective*. Paper presented at the 3rd National Outlook Symposium on Crime in Australia, Mapping the Boundaries of Australia's Criminal Justice System convened by the Australian Institute of Criminology, Canberra, 22–23 March 1999.

Degenhardt, L. and Topp, L. (2003) '"Crystal meth" use among polydrug users in Sydney's dance party subculture: characteristics, use patterns and associated harms', *International Journal of Drug Policy*, 14: 17–24.

Duff, C. (2003) 'Drugs and youth cultures: Is Australia experiencing the "normalization" of adolescent drug use?' *Journal of Youth Studies*, 6: 433–46.

Ennett, S., Bailey, S. and Federman, E. (1999) 'Social network characteristics associated with risky behaviors among runaway and homeless youth', *Journal of Health and Social Behavior*, 40 (March): 63–78.

Flom, P., Friedman, S., Kottiri, J., Neaigus, A., Curtis, R., Des Jarlais, D., Sandoval, M. and Zenilman, J. (2001) 'Stigmatized drug use, sexual partner concurrency, and other sex risk network and behavior characteristics of 18- to 24-year-old youth in a high-risk neighborhood', *Sexually Transmitted Diseases*, 28: 598–607.

Friedman, S., Flom, P., Kottiri, B., Neaigus, A., Sandoval, M., Curtis, R., Zenilman, J. and Des Jarlais, D. (2001) 'Prevalence and correlates of anal sex with men among young adult women in an inner city minority neighborhood', *AIDS*, 15: 2057–60.

Friedman, S., Friedmann, P., Telles, P., Bastos, F., Bueno, R., Mesquita, F. and Des Jarlais, D. (1998a) 'New injectors and HIV risk', in G. Stimson, D. Des Jarlais and A. Ball (eds) *Drug Injecting and HIV Infection*, London: UCL Press, pp. 76–90.

Friedman, S., Jose, B., Stepherson, B., Neaigus, A., Goldstein, M., Mota, P., Curtis, R. and Ildefonso, G. (1998b) 'Multiple racial/ethnic subordination and HIV among drug injectors', in M. Singer (ed.) *The Political Economy of AIDS*, New York: Baywood.

Gilman, M. (1994) 'Football and drugs: two cultures clash', *The International Journal of Drug Policy*, 5(1). Online. Available HTTP: <http://www.drugtext.org/library/articles/945108.htm> (accessed 26 February 2004).

Government of Bangladesh (2000) *Report on the Second Expanded HIV Surveillance, 1999–2000*, Bangladesh: Government of Bangladesh/UNAIDS.

Grob, C. and Dobkin de Rios, M. (1992) 'Adolescent drug use in cross-cultural perspective', *Journal of Drug Issues*, 22: 121–38.

Hong, S. and Shepherd, M. (1996) 'Psychosocial and demographic predictors of pediatric psychotropic medication use', *American Journal of Health-System Pharmacy*, 53: 1934–9.

Human Rights Watch (2000) 'United States: punishment and prejudice: racial disparities in the criminal justice system', *Human Rights Watch* 12, No. 2(G), May. Online. Available HTTP: <http://www.hrw.org/reports/2000/usa/> (accessed 26 February 2004).

International Crisis Group (2003) 'Youth in central Asia: losing the new generation', *ICG Asia Report* No. 66, October 31.

Jeffrey, D., Klein, A. and King, L. (2001) *Report to the EMCDDA by the REITOX National Focal Point: United Kingdom Drug Situation, 2001*, Lisbon: DrugScope and the European Monitoring Centre for Drugs and Drug Dependency.

Jelsma, M. (2003) 'Drugs in the UN system: the unwritten history of the 1998 United Nations General Assembly Special Session on drugs', *International Journal of Drug Policy*, 14: 181–95.

Johnston, L., O'Malley, P. and Bachman, J. (2003a) 'Monitoring the Future: national results on adolescent drug use. Overview of key findings, 2002' (NIH Publication No. 03-5374), Bethesda, MD: National Institute on Drug Abuse. Online. Available HTTP: http://www.monitoringthefuture.org/pubs/monographs/overview 2002.pdf (accessed 30 May 2004).

Johnston, L., O'Malley, P. and Bachman, J. (2003b) 'Demographic subgroup trends for various licit and illicit drugs, 1975–2002' (Monitoring the Future Occasional Paper No. 59), Ann Arbor, MI: Institute for Social Research. Online. Available HTTP <http://www.monitoringthefuture.org/pubs/occpapers/occ59.pdf> (accessed 30 May 2004).

Johnston, L., O'Malley, P., Bachman, J. and Schulenberg, J. (2004) 'Monitoring the Future national results on adolescent drug use. Overview of key findings, 2003' (NIH Publication No. 04-5506), Bethesda, MD: National Institute on Drug Abuse. Online. Available HTTP: http://www.monitoringthefuture.org/pubs/monographs/ overview2003.pdf (accessed 30 May 2004).

Kalunta-Crumpton, A. (2003) 'Problematic drug use among "invisible" ethnic minorities', *Journal of Substance Use*, 8: 170–5.

Kane, J.L. (2001) 'How Effective is the Current Drug Policy?' United States Senior District Judge, speech presented at University of Denver Faculty Forum, May.

Kreft, I.G.G. and Brown, J.H. (eds) (1998) 'Zero effects of drug prevention programs: issues and solutions', *Evaluation Review*, 22: 3–14.

Krohn, F. and Suazo, F. (1995) 'Contemporary urban music: controversial messages in hip-hop and rap lyrics', *International Society for General Semantics*. Online. Available HTTP: <http://www.sistahspace.com/nommo/mv13.html> (accessed 26 February 2004).

Lin, K.-M. and Poland, R. (2000) 'Ethnicity, culture, and psychopharmacology', *Back to Psychopharmacology – The Fourth Generation of Progress*. Online. Available HTTP: <http://www.acnp.org/g4/GN401000184/CH180.html> (accessed 1 April 2004).

National Institute on Drug Abuse (NIDA) (2003) *Drug Use among Racial/Ethnic Minorities* (NIH Publication No. 03-3888), Bethesda, MD: US Department of Health and Human Services/National Institutes of Health.

Parker, H. (2003) 'Pathology or modernity? Rethinking risk factor analyses of young drug users', *Dependency Research and Theory*, 11: 141–4.

Parker, H., Aldridge, J. and Measham, F. (1998) *Illegal Leisure: The Normalization of Adolescent Drug Use*, London: Routledge.

Reinarman, C. and Duskin, C. (1992) 'Dominant ideology and drugs in the media', *International Journal on Drug Policy*, 3: 6–15.

Rivera, L. (2002) 'Youth subcultures in Puerto Rico, an observation. Puerto Rico.com, January', *The Atabey Project*, Online. Available HTTP: www.nutslapper.com (accessed 9 January 2004).

Rojanaphruk, P. (2004) 'No quick fixes', *The Nation* (Thailand), February 6. Online. Available HTTP: <http://www.nationmultimedia.com/page.arcview.php3?clid=26&id=93610&usrsess=1> (accessed 10 February 2004).

Rose, T. (1994) *Black Noise: Rap Music and Black Culture in Contemporary America*, New Hampshire: University Press of New England.

Seppälä, P. and Salasuo, M. (n.d.) 'Drugs and rave culture'. Online. Available HTTP: <http://www.paihdelinkki.fi/english/infobank/400_drug_line/462e.htm> (accessed 26 February 2004).

Sherman, S. and Latkin, C. (2002) 'Drug users' involvement in the drug economy: implication for harm reduction and HIV prevention programs', *Journal of Urban Health: Bulletin of the New York Academy of Medicine*, 79: 266–77.

Soul Beat Africa (2003) 'Effect of culture and environment on the behaviour of Namibian youth', *Soul Beat Africa*. Online. Available HTTP: <http://www.comminit.com/strategicthinking/st2003/thinking-154.html> (accessed 13 October 2003).

Swaim, R., Beauvais, F., Chavez, E. and Oetting, E. (1997) 'The effect of school dropout rates on estimates of adolescent substance use among three racial/ethnic groups', *American Journal of Public Health*, 87: 51–5.

Zito, J., Safer, D., DosReis, S., Gardner, J., Magder, L., Soeken, K., Bole, M., Lynch, F. and Riddle, M. (2003) 'Psychotropic practice patterns for youth: a 10-year perspective', *Archives of Pediatrics and Adolescent Medicine*, 157: 17–25.

Part II

Young people, sex and drugs

Chapter 5

Young people, sexual practice and meanings

Deborah Keys, Doreen Rosenthal and Marian Pitts

Young people are not an homogeneous group – a fact obscured by concepts such as 'adolescence', which imply common experiences or at the least common characteristics and predispositions. Moreover, young people's sexuality and sexual behaviour need to be located within the broader context of their lives. Sexuality and its expressions do not occur outside of culture, despite their seeming naturalness due to the fact that they involve the body. The relationship between culture and sex is complex. Sexuality and sexual behaviour are not simply shaped in response to dominant and/or subcultural meanings and their manifestations but in part develop *out of* sexual discourses as expressed through social interaction, the media and consumer capitalism.

In spite of reporting on a number of negative outcomes here, young people's sexuality and sexual behaviour involve more than negative possibilities or risks (see for example, Irvine 1994, Aggleton and Campbell 2000). Sexuality is both a source and expression of crucial and potentially pleasurable and positive aspects of a young person's identity. However, the terms 'young people' and 'sex' usually occur in relation to some kind of problem. Indeed, the fact that young people are sexual at all seems to arouse concern in many cultures. But is there only cause for concern? What are the sexual practices of young people and what are the meanings attached to them?

Sexual behaviour

This chapter looks at the links between sexual behaviour, sexual well-being and sexual vulnerability within a framework that stresses the positive potential of young people as sexual beings. While we consider condom use, we do not look more broadly at other forms of contraception or reproductive health. The extent to which young people are vulnerable to contracting HIV/AIDS and other sexually transmissible infections, experiencing an unwanted pregnancy or suffering sexual harm varies enormously according to the personal and contextual factors noted throughout this book.

How behaviour and its outcomes are evaluated – as problematic, acceptable or valued – does of course also vary according to the sexual meanings individuals subscribe to and the sexual cultures they inhabit. For example, wanted and unwanted pregnancies to single and coupled young women are often conflated under the heading 'teen pregnancy' and seen by definition as problems. However, the experiences and likely outcomes for a single, pregnant 13-year-old living in poverty and without family support and a 19-year-old living with a partner and enjoying a planned pregnancy are very different.

An overriding issue is that of gender. Gender differences are deeply structured, underpinning sexual cultures and informing sexual meanings in various ways. A UNAIDS study of sex and youth in seven developing countries found that, despite differences between and within countries and regions, there was overall a similar differential in cultural understandings of young men's and young women's sexuality (UNAIDS 1999). The study found that across virtually all cultures, young men are seen to be sexual beings and encouraged to become sexually active, while young women are expected to embrace abstinence (Dowsett *et al.* 1998). Such understandings continue to inform sexual cultures and meanings in many, if not most, locations.

Sexual initiation

We need to view the issue of age of sexual 'debut' – here referring to first penile–vaginal intercourse (a point taken up later) – in light of the historical picture. The decrease in age of initiation, particularly in developed countries, can be seen as a swing of the pendulum rather than a new occurrence. Prior to the twentieth century early marriage and initiation were the norm in many countries. The gap between the age of puberty and age of marriage has never been greater in the West – a situation that almost guarantees that more sex will occur between those who are young and unmarried.

The importance of culture

Despite moves towards a more global youth culture, often accompanied by a shift to Western individualism, traditional cultures remain extremely influential in relation to the sexual behaviour of young people in non-Western countries (Caldwell *et al.* 1998). For example, age of sexual initiation tends to be later (although generally dropping) in Asian countries where the continuing value of female virginity is predicated on earlier concerns with controlling inheritance and the importance of class.

While a traditional commitment to female pre-marital virginity may result in lower overall rates of unwanted pregnancy, it can also result in less use of contraception by those who do have sex and serious consequences for those who become pregnant. A Korean study (Tai-hwan, Hee and Sung-nam 1999) found that while contraception was shunned by many young women as being at odds with their self-image as virtuous, sex did still take place, sometimes resulting in pregnancy – a shameful experience for those who had seen themselves as respectable.

Conversely, in some parts of Africa the historical importance of fertility means that although sexually active unmarried young women may have been punished in the past, the level of shame associated with such behaviour is generally lower than in Asian countries (Caldwell *et al.* 1998). Clearly, as Dehne and Riedner (2001) among others have observed, young people around the world may experience similar physical changes as they grow older, but the way in which these are interpreted, and the social and legal proscriptions attending them, vary tremendously. Cultural factors are subject to change but the process is one of assimilation and incorporation rather than disconnection or rupture.

Pushes and pulls

Social factors associated with age of sexual initiation include gender, class, ethnicity and family, peer and institutional influence (Rosenthal, Smith and de Visser 1999), all of which interact with personal characteristics such as perception of oneself in relation to peers, views on gender, and degree of desire for autonomy. In short, becoming sexually active, either as a result of a cognitive evaluation of the pros and cons or as an unmeditated spontaneous response, occurs in a complex environment in which competing factors exert influence. There are pushes – both biological (earlier puberty) and cultural (for example, the sexualization of children and young teens by the media and consumer culture) – and pulls (increase in the age of marriage and social censure). These factors will weigh differently for young men and women.

Variations and trends

Despite considerable differences in age of initiation between countries (UNAIDS 2002), overall, young men tend to experience sexual debut at a younger age than young women (Population Information Program 2001, Singh *et al.* 2000, Youn 2001). There are of course exceptions. In a number of countries (for example, Cameroon, the USA, Australia and Britain) the average age of initiation is almost the same for males and females. In a minority of cases, including countries as diverse as Finland and Nigeria, a greater percentage of young women than young men have experienced intercourse before they turned 15 (UNAIDS 2002). While disparity in age of partners, in particular with the male being older than the female, suggests inequality in the power relationship, increasing young women's vulnerability, a common age of initiation does not necessarily reflect equality.

Overwhelmingly, a young woman's good reputation remains linked to restraint in sexual behaviour while that of a young man does not (Rosenthal and Smith 1997).

Gender is not the only significant differentiating factor within countries, there are also differences in relation to ethnicity and sexual orientation. For example, many US studies report differences in age of first sex between African-Americans, whites and Latinos, with black males being at the early end of the continuum (for example, Grunbaum *et al.* 2002, Cooksey, Mott and Neubauer 2002). In some studies, early sexual initiation has also been found to be associated with gay, lesbian or bisexual self-identification in the USA (Garofalo *et al.* 1998, Rosario *et al.* 1999).

The heterogeneous nature of young people and their circumstances mean that we cannot generalize about age of initiation. The median age of first sexual experience ranges from 15 to 22 (UNICEF, UNAIDS and WHO 2002) although in certain countries initiation may be very common at the extremes of the category we call young people. A recent large survey of children and young people in the poorest sections of Zambia's capital reported that one quarter of 10-year-olds said they had already had sex (UNAIDS 2000). At the other extreme, most young people in China experience first sexual intercourse after turning 20 (UNAIDS 2000).

While the trend worldwide has been towards earlier sexual initiation, in some places this seems to be changing. A major US study has reported a reduction over the last ten years in the percentage of students who first had sex before the age of 13 from 10.2 to 6.6 per cent (CDC 2003). The average age of first sex among urban youth in Uganda rose by two years between 1989 and 1995 (Asiimwe-Okiror *et al.* in Population Information Program 2001) and in the UK there are signs that the trend towards a decreasing age of initiation for young women may be stabilizing (Wellings *et al.* 2001). It has been posited that the trend is reversing in some countries as a result of HIV/AIDS and prevention campaigns (UNAIDS 2000).

Early initiation and increased vulnerability

Findings vary greatly but we can conclude that in many places/cases a relationship exists between early sexual debut and greater vulnerability. Some studies have found that the younger the individual's age of initiation, the greater the number of likely partners (UNICEF, UNAIDS and WHO 2002, Coker *et al.* 1994, O'Donnell, O'Donnell and Stueve 2001, Rissel *et al.* 2003), the less likelihood of regular condom use (UNICEF, UNAIDS and WHO 2002, Coker *et al.* 1994), and the greater the chance of pregnancy (Wellings *et al.* 2001, Coker *et al.* 1994, O'Donnell, O'Donnell and Stueve 2001, Zavodny 2001), contracting a sexually transmitted infection (STI) (Coker *et al.* 1994, Rissel *et al.* 2003) or HIV (UNAIDS 2000). Certainly, young women are physiologically more vulnerable to STIs and HIV infection than older women (Population Information Program 2001, UNICEF, UNAIDS and WHO 2002). However, it may be that early initiators were at greater risk primarily because of the extended period of sexually active youth, rather than any common proclivities or behaviours among those who start young.

The fact that first sexual intercourse is rarely planned has led to concern that young people, particularly young women, may be at greater risk of STIs and HIV infection, in addition to unwanted pregnancy, as contraception may not be used. However, some recent studies in developed countries found that although average age of first vaginal intercourse has dropped over the last 30 years, condom use at first sex has increased substantially (Grunbaum *et al.* 2002, Wellings *et al.* 2001, Rissel *et al.* 2003).

Early initiation, however, is more likely to involve coercion (Abma, Driscoll and Moore 1998, Cáceres, Marin and Hudes 2000, Alan Guttmacher Institute 1999). Only 28 per cent of young women in Jamaica say they were willing partners at sexual initiation (UNICEF, UNAIDS and WHO 2002). Women whose first partner was seven or more years older than themselves were more than twice as likely as those whose first partner was the same age or younger to rate the experience as low on the degree of 'wantedness' scale (Abma, Driscoll and Moore 1998). There seems to be an ongoing effect on sexual health in some situations. For example, in Lima it has been reported that those who are coerced at initiation are more likely to experience an STI at a later date (Cáceres, Marin and Hudes 2000). These findings indicate that in some circumstances early sexual initiation, especially for young women, holds particular risks.

However, early sexual initiation is not necessarily a problem in itself. Rather, lack of information, education and/or support for those in their early teens may lead to unwelcome outcomes for those who experience an early sexual debut. The association between early initiation and drug use, delinquency and smoking (identified in many studies as risk factors) may reflect one aspect of more positive proclivities towards independent, non-conforming ideas and a drive towards autonomy (as reported in others). Labelling young people's sexuality as just another risk-taking behaviour (Jessor and Jessor 1977) obscures the positive side of an urge to experience and experiment – crucial precursors to growth.

Sexual partners

The possibility of positive sexual experiences is linked to *whom* young people take as sexual partners, not because of any inherent individual qualities but either because of existing structural inequality (for example, age or socio-economic) or the prevalence of particular practices amongst particular groups of individuals. In this respect, age differentials and the nature of the relationship are particularly salient.

Age differentials between partners

Age differentials between partners commonly affect sexual health outcomes, with those of both sexes more vulnerable when partnered by older men. In addition to being more likely to involve coercion, sex between older men and younger women is associated with more pregnancies and greater risk of HIV in some circumstances. A woman whose partner is seven or more years older is also less likely than other women to use contraceptives at first intercourse (Abma, Driscoll and Moore 1998). The fact that young women in sub-Saharan Africa are almost twice as likely as young men to contract HIV/AIDS has, in part, been attributed to the prevalence of sexual relationships between young women and older men (UNAIDS/WHO 2002).

A recent Australian study found that young men who have sex with men were significantly more likely than same-sex attracted young women to be initiated by a partner five or more years older (Grulich *et al.* 2003). Young men are also vulnerable to sexual coercion by older partners. For example, around 7.5 per cent of 314 young men surveyed in a Sri Lankan study reported being sexually coerced by an older male when they were 13 or younger (Shanler *et al.* 1998).

Multiple partners

Some young people have multiple partners, either as a result of 'one-night stands' or serial monogamy, while others only have sex with long-term regular partners. Of course, the greater the number of partners, the greater the possibility of exposure to an STI or HIV. Generally, young men are more likely than young women to have sex with casual partners and to have more sexual partners (Moore and Rosenthal 1993). One-third of young men in a recent Kenyan study reported having more than ten sexual partners before marriage (UNAIDS 2000) while the US Youth Risk Behavior Survey of school students (2001) found that 14 per cent (both males and females) said they had had four or more sex partners (Grunbaum *et al.* 2002).

Early marriage

Not all young people have sex outside marriage. While the issues are very different for those who are having sanctioned sex, young married women are particularly at risk because they are more likely to be married to older men and experience the increased vulnerability to HIV/STIs for those reasons outlined above. While pregnancy may be a desired outcome, there are increased risks to reproductive health for young women. The leading cause of death for women between the ages of 15 and 19 is related to pregnancy, childbirth and unsafe abortion (United Nations in UNFPA 2003). Girls under age 15 are five times as likely to die in childbirth as those in their twenties

(Reborças in UNFPA 2003). Those living in South Asia and some parts of Africa are particularly likely to marry at a young age. Seventy-six per cent of young women in Niger are married by the age of 18 and in Nepal almost 20 per cent marry before the age of 15 (UNICEF, UNAIDS and WHO 2002). In many countries, teenage sexual intercourse predominantly occurs outside marriage for men but largely within marriage for women (Singh *et al.* 2000).

Trading sex

Young people trade sex legally and illegally, by choice or necessity, independently and under contract, and in situations ranging from the exploitative (such as sex trafficking) to those in which they are in a position to exert control. The continuum of sex for exchange includes the very different practices of 'survival sex', 'transactional sex' and 'commercial sex'. Transactional sex, where young women are having sex with older men in exchange for money or gifts is common in many places in Africa (UNAIDS/WHO 2002, Silberschmidt and Rasch 2001, Buve *et al.* 2002, Panos Institute 2001, Luke and Kurz 2002). This practice, often motivated by young women's desire to get an education or otherwise improve their opportunities in life can backfire, as they are often entering into relationships in which they are likely to have little power to negotiate safer sex practices.

With regard to commercial sex, young people are both clients and sex workers. Most sex workers start work when they are young and the level of autonomy they possess, the direness or otherwise of their situation, and the legislative and regulatory environment will impact upon how vulnerable they are to sexual harm such as rape and unprotected sex. The estimated one million children who are forced into the sex trade every year (UNICEF, UNAIDS and WHO 2002) are particularly at risk.

In some cultures, young men are traditionally initiated into sex by sex workers. However, this is beginning to change in some countries. In Thailand, where growing HIV prevalence led to an intensive HIV/AIDS campaign and young women are increasingly likely to engage in sex before marriage, young men are less likely to lose their virginity through sex with sex workers (Van Landingham 2002).

Sexual practices

It is hard to generalize about how many young people are sexually active other than to say that for most people sexual activity begins in their youth. The percentage of those who report ever having had sex varies from less than 2 per cent of never married 15–19 year-old young men in Sri Lanka (UNAIDS 2000) to 48.5 per cent of age 10–24 male students in the USA (Grunbaum *et al.* 2002). In the Ivory Coast, 73 per cent of women report sexual activity (Population Reference Bureau 2001) while much lower numbers of unmarried women of the same age reported being sexually active in the Philippines (UNAIDS 2000). Young women in the Philippines may well have been reluctant to report their sexual activities, resulting in under reporting. However, these findings indicate not only the existence of powerful cultural imperatives, but also the strong possibility that these imperatives may result in lower levels of sexual activity among young women than elsewhere.

Neither is it wise to generalize about the frequency with which young people are having sex. What it is possible to say, however, is that sexual initiation does not necessarily translate into an ongoing active sex life (Moore and Rosenthal 1993). For some, especially those not in a relationship, sexual relations may be sporadic. In 2001, only one-third of young people surveyed for the US Youth Risk Behaviour Survey reported having had sexual intercourse during the three months preceding the survey (Grunbaum *et al.* 2002).

Cultural context

There is no doubt that young people and sex is contested terrain. The anxieties and constraints surrounding the sexual behaviour of young people indicate that adults regard them as sexual beings, but they also reflect the predominant adult view that young people are not ready to express their sexual feelings or desires. As a result, young people often find themselves having to establish their sexual identities in a realm of competing messages. The USA, seen by many as the source of a globalized youth culture that promotes sexual freedom, has a government with a clear moral agenda expressed through a funding bias to abstinence-only sex education, despite the fact that there is no evidence that this approach is the most effective (Kirby 2002). The USA also has one of the highest rates of teenage pregnancy in the Western world, despite a recent downturn (Darroch, Singh and Frost 2001, Kirby 2001, Alan Guttmacher Institute 2002, Darroch and Singh 1999).

Even at the level of the local, sexual cultures compete. They are also in flux as sexual meanings are constantly adapted and reformed. Living within rapidly changing sexual cultures may increase vulnerability, as conflicting meanings come into play. Moving between sexual cultures also involves negotiation. This may be particularly the case for young people leaving developing countries with strict proscriptions regarding sexual behaviour amongst unmarried youth for Western cities where adult surveillance may be minimal and sex is less proscribed. Lack of education in sex and relationships is likely to render such students more vulnerable to negative sexual and reproductive outcomes. Young same-sex attracted individuals experiencing Western gay, lesbian (or queer) cultures organized around a positive sense of sexual self may find it difficult to reconcile the conflicting sexual cultures upon returning home.

Attraction and identity: the fluidity of experience

Fluidity of sexual attraction and uncertainty regarding sexual identity are not only the province of the young, but they seem to be particularly salient for those in the early years of sexual experience. Sexual preference regarding gender of partner is variously gauged according to sexual attraction, sexual activity and sexual identification. Despite this, it is clear that a considerable proportion of young people do not fit the expectation of an undeviating heterosexuality. Student surveys have found levels of exclusive heterosexuality ranging from 71 to 95 per cent (Amirkanian, Tiunov and Kelly 2001, Edgardh, 2002, Smith *et al.* 2003). A recent Australian study (Smith *et al.* 2003) found that just over 5 per cent of secondary students reported some attraction to those of the same sex or that they were unsure, while a study of homeless youth in the same country reported that 22.5 per cent were attracted to those of the same sex to some degree, although only 12 per cent identified as gay, homosexual, lesbian or bisexual and 5.2 per cent were unsure (Keys 2003). These findings indicate something of the complexity of sexual identity, and demonstrate the consequent difficulties in drawing straightforward comparisons and conclusions. The longitudinal study of homeless young people also found the percentage of those changing identification after twelve months was high (12.5 per cent).

Same-sex sanctions and sexual health

Differing sexual cultures involving social, religious and legal sanctions affect both the meanings associated with same-sex attraction and sexual practices and the level of occurrence. In a few countries, there has been a move towards greater tolerance, if not whole-hearted acceptance of same sex relations.

However, continuing sanctions mean that maintaining a positive understanding of one's sexual self and sexual health more generally is harder to achieve for young people who are same-sex attracted. One San Franciscan study found that a greater acceptance of gay or bisexual identity was associated with safer sex practices for 13 to 17-year-old same-sex attracted males (Waldo *et al.* 2000).

There is evidence that some same-sex attracted young people in non-Western countries are adopting Western versions of gay identity (for example) at a time when young people in the West may be increasingly reluctant to adopt such identities (Reynolds 2002). For example, in the Philippines, the terms 'gay' and 'lesbian' have been incorporated into the language, however the specificity of local sexual cultures and identities makes such adoptions less than simple (Tan 2001). In Asia, where aspects of globalization, such as social and economic transformations and merging local and Western discourses and cultures are contributing to rapidly changing sexual cultures (Jackson 2001), there may be gains in regard to freedom to enjoy sexual experiences and, unless concomitant attitudinal and educational change occurs, losses in regard to sexual health for young people.

Multiple motivations

Young people embark on sexual careers for many reasons, ranging from the affective to the financial. Gender differences are significant influences on meaning, with males often more likely to cite pleasure, desire and physical satisfaction and females, love, intimacy or desire for a close relationship (Dowsett *et al.* 1998, Moore and Rosenthal 1993). This may well be related to cultural expectations around gender and sexuality. However, some studies have revealed evidence of gender convergence, for example, among middle-class Anglo-Australian youth (Moore and Rosenthal 1993). Differences in motivation have also been found between those young women who have sex earlier (peers having sex, curiosity and feeling grown up) and those who are initiated later (love and attraction) (Rosenthal *et al.* 2001). Young women have also been found to feel less satisfied after first intercourse, or to regret it more often, than do young men (Rosenthal and Smith 1997, Wellings *et al.* 2001, Dickson *et al.* 1998).

Towards a broader definition of sex

Having started with a discussion of penile–vaginal intercourse as the act that designates sexual initiation, as defined in most studies, we would like to undercut that position by stressing the need to define sex more broadly. Mutual masturbation and oral and anal sex must be recognized as important elements of sexual experience. Even from a health perspective such a position is warranted, as some of these practices (when unprotected) have the potential to result in STI or HIV infection. There are also important implications for education. In the USA, despite the $50 billion of federal funds spent per annum on abstinence education, there is little consensus among young people or educators as to whether oral or anal sex qualify as abstinence (Remez 2000). One study found that 59 per cent of students surveyed did not class oral sex as sex (Sanders and Reinisch in Remez 2000). In Mauritius, penetration up to the point of pain is not considered to result in loss of virginity for young women (Weiss, Whelan and Gupta 2000). Both virginity and abstinence are social constructs currently under revision in many societies.

Oral and anal sex

Little is known about the prevalence of oral and anal sex among young people, probably in part because of the difficulty in obtaining funding and consent for such research (Remez 2000). This is especially so in relation to heterosexual youth. In recent years, there has been greater recognition of anal sex as heterosexual practice. Like oral sex, it is now seen by many as just part of their sexual repertoire. The finding that young people are enjoying a wider sexual repertoire than before (Dowsett *et al.* 1998) may in part be attributable to more specific questions being asked along with a greater willingness to report, but Moore and Rosenthal (1993), among others, have argued that the generality of such findings suggests that young people *are* becoming more sexually adventurous.

Most studies report that oral sex is more common than anal sex. For instance, over 50 per cent of 15- to 19-year-old Australians have experienced heterosexual oral sex, whereas only 4 per cent have participated in heterosexual anal sex. The occurrence of anal sex varies greatly across and within countries, with studies finding anything between 2 and 39 per cent of various youth populations reporting participating in anal sex (Amirkanian, Tiunov and Kelly 2001, Edgardh 2002, Stanton *et al.* 1994). These figures relate predominantly but not exclusively to heterosexual-identified samples.

A study of Australian youth experiencing homelessness found that 25 per cent of homeless 16-year-old men and women reported having engaged in anal sex (Rosenthal, Moore and Buzwell 1994), a finding that demonstrates the importance of considering sexual cultures at the level of milieu in relation to practice. That homelessness is commonly associated with higher than average levels of drug use, which may impede safer sex practices, makes this situation particularly worrying (Mallet *et al.* 2003).

Heterosexual anal sex has long been posited as a contributing factor in the spread of HIV in sub-Saharan Africa (Brody and Potterat 2003). In heterosexual sex, anal sex is sometimes used as a way to protect a woman's virginity (as proved by an intact hymen) and prevent pregnancy (Weiss, Whelan and Gupta 2000) rather than solely for the purpose of sexual pleasure.

Sexual safety

Sexual safety encompasses freedom from coercion, exploitation, sexual ill-health and unwanted pregnancy. It also paves the way for positive sexual possibilities. Despite some encouraging reports from particular locations (including Thailand, Zambia, Brazil and Uganda), more than 6,000 15- to 24-year-olds around the world are infected with HIV each day and studies reveal that the vast majority of young people do not know how HIV is transmitted or how to protect themselves (UNICEF, UNAIDS and WHO 2002). As recently as 1999, 95 per cent of young women in Bangladesh did not know how to protect themselves against HIV/AIDS (Population Information Program 2001) and this in a country in which another study reported that 88 per cent of unmarried, urban males had engaged in sexual activity (presumably not all with each other) by 18 years of age (UNICEF, UNAIDS and WHO 2002). Even less awareness exists regarding other sexually transmitted infections. Rapid increases in rates of chlamydia, syphilis and gonorrhoea in the UK (UNAIDS/WHO 2002, Panchaud *et al.* 2000) indicate that it is not only those in developing countries who are engaging in risky behaviour.

Impediments to sexual health

In addition to lack of knowledge, gaps between knowledge and practice and unavailability of services combine with broader cultural and contextual factors to affect young people's sexual health. There is a general recognition that even those who do have knowledge are vulnerable to infection; considerable gaps exist between knowledge and practice.

In the past, research has concentrated on possible individual and developmental explanations for this. More recently, however, there has been a growing focus on contextual factors. Unavailability of condoms or lack of access to clinics and information are only the most obvious impediments. Many health campaigns attempt to foster better communication between sexual partners but communication regarding contraception occurs within sexual cultures. Patriarchy and tradition, particularly in relation to double standards around gender, can result in levels of inequality and stigma that render such 'negotiation' all but impossible (Aggleton 1996). In Dar es Salaam, young women engaging in transactional sex with 'sugar daddies' are sexually active in a culture where only sex workers can, without aspersion or censure, request that a condom be used (Silberschmidt and Rasch 2001).

Another important contextual factor is that of financial pressure (see, for example, Bohmer and Kirumira 2000). In regions where HIV prevalence is high, gender inequality can prove fatal (Gupta 2003). Desperate socio-economic situations can lead to a lack of ability to ensure safe sex. AIDS orphans and young people living in situations of conflict or population displacement are particularly vulnerable.

Levels of condom use during anal sex are particularly worrying. Of 15- to 22-year-old San Franciscan men who had had anal sex with men, 41 per cent reported having unprotected anal sex within six months prior to being interviewed (Valleroy *et al.* in Futterman 2003). In another study, more than 72 per cent of young Latino men who had sex with men said they had had unprotected anal intercourse (UNICEF, UNAIDS and WHO 2002). Other studies have shown increased levels of unprotected anal sex among young men (for example, Strathdee *et al.* 2000). It has been suggested by some that this may be related to optimism in relation to better anti-retroviral treatment (Dilley, Woods and McFarlane 1997). Because heterosexuals are rarely a target population for health messages about safe anal sex, it is likely that many are having such sex without condoms.

Unwanted pregnancy

Unwanted pregnancy is the other unwelcome outcome of intercourse without contraception. In those countries where public health policies adopt a comprehensive approach, birth rates among the young tend to be lower. In the Netherlands, for example, the birth rate for the under 20s was 6.2 per thousand, while in the USA it was 52.2 (UNICEF 2001). Undoubtedly many teenage pregnancies have negative impacts, particularly on the young women involved. Whether they resolve in a birth or abortion, the possibility of poor medical or psychological outcomes or negative social ramifications exists.

Cultural factors, such as level of stigma, and social factors, such as legal status of abortion, along with broader social, economic and political circumstances will affect the likelihood of a positive or negative outcome. However, we must never forget that for many young people a conception may be planned or welcome. Even amongst those who become pregnant in less than optimal circumstances, the possibility of increased self-esteem and enhancement of life through positive experiences of parenting exists. There is, moreover, some debate as to whether poor social outcomes, such as poverty, for young mothers and their children are the result of the pregnancy itself or reflect continuance of a situation that was likely to be ongoing in any case (Furstenberg 1998).

Sexual coercion

Sexual coercion, from unwanted persuasion to rape, and involving regular partners, acquaintances and strangers, is also an issue. As with condom use, there can be a considerable gap between knowledge (for example of what constitutes pressure) and practice (Rosenthal 1997). Thirty-nine per cent of young women in a recent South African study said they had been coerced into sex (UNAIDS 2002). Male college students in a US study were as likely to have experienced sexual coercion (though not physical force) as female students (Larimer *et al.* 1999). In some circumstances, rapid economic and social change can contribute to changes in sexual cultures that include more frequent and diverse forms of sexual violence (Dowsett *et al.* 1998, UNAIDS/WHO 2002).

Positive possibilities

A research and practice focus on sexual health problems has meant that the positive possibilities of young people's sexuality have been largely ignored. These aspects include having a sense of control over one's sexual experiences/sexual autonomy; the opportunity to express (and have recognized) one's sexuality/sexual identity; the ability to derive pleasure from one's sexual life; the ability to form positive sexual relationships; and the opportunity to practise adult roles, including relationship building, which may enhance self-esteem and more general feelings of autonomy.

Overall, young people and sexual pleasure remains an under-researched field, and young people's sexual pleasure is largely unaddressed by sex education or society more generally.

Conclusions

In recent years, there have been some positive shifts in relation to young people and sex. In some countries, these have involved recognition that sexual expression does not inevitably lead to sexual or reproductive problems or disasters. An increasing number of young people live in cultures where the censure of same-sex attraction or expression is abating. To various degrees, changing gender relations have brought about a climate in which young women and indeed young men are less prepared to sit back and accept what is given.

Young people *do* have agency in relation to the way they express their sexuality, both through sexual practices and the adoption of sexual identities. However, this agency is curtailed or assisted by circumstances often outside their direct control. As a group, young people have little political power and are largely excluded from decisions that affect their lives, sexual and other-wise. They are generally regarded as developmentally incapable, wilfully uncooperative or as passive victims; in Aggleton and Warwick's (1997) terms as 'mad', 'bad' or 'sad'.

Young people usually develop sexual meanings and make decisions regarding sexual practices and sexual identity within environments that are unlikely to be conducive to the development of positive, healthy sexual selves. 'Enabling environments' (Aggleton and Campbell 1999) that recognize young people as sexual beings optimize the possibility of good sexual and reproductive health. In such settings a young person's sexuality is viewed as a positive attribute, there is relatively open communication about sexual matters, and the education and services that make it possible for young people to reduce their levels of vulnerability to adverse outcomes are provided.

Considering the complexity of factors in play around young people's sexuality and sexual practice allows us to move away from the notion of adolescent risk-takers and embrace the idea of young people as sexual subjects. It also allows us to recognize that sexual behaviour that has hitherto been regarded as problematic can have various outcomes – both positive and negative. Such a move paves the way for more progressive programmatic responses to sexual and reproductive health.

References

Abma, J., Driscoll, A. and Moore, K. (1998) 'Young women's degree of control over first intercourse: An exploratory analysis', *Family Planning Perspectives*, 30: 12–18.

Aggleton, P. (1996) 'Sexual practices, sexually transmitted diseases and AIDS amongst young people', in *Seminario Internacional sobre Avances en Salud Reproductiva y Sexualidad*, Mexico: El Colegio de Mexico.

Aggleton, P. and Campbell, C. (1999) *Paper 4: HIV/AIDS policy issues relating to youth*, Montebello, Canada: Health Canada/UNAIDS International Policy Dialogue on AIDS.

Aggleton, P. and Campbell, C. (2000) 'Working with young people: Towards an agenda for sexual health (Summary)', *Sexual and Relationship Therapy*, 15: 283–96.

Aggleton, P. and Warwick, I. (1997) 'Young people, sexuality, HIV and AIDS education', in L. Sherr (ed.) *AIDS and Adolescents*, Amsterdam: Harwood Academic, pp. 79–90.

Alan Guttmacher Institute (1999) *Teen Sex and Pregnancy: Facts in Brief*, New York and Washington: Alan Guttmacher Institute.

Alan Guttmacher Institute (2002) *Teen Pregnancy: Trends and Lessons Learned. Issues in Brief* (Series, No.1), New York: Alan Guttmacher Institute.

Amirkanian, Y., Tiunov, D. and Kelly, J. (2001) 'Risk factors for HIV and other sexually transmitted diseases among adolescents in St. Petersburg, Russia', *Family Planning Perspectives*, 33: 106–12.

Bohmer, L. and Kirumira, E.K. (2000) 'Socio-economic context and the sexual behaviour of Ugandan out of school youth', *Culture, Health and Sexuality*, 2: 269–85.

Brody, S. and Potterat, J. (2003) 'Assessing the role of anal intercourse in the epidemiology of AIDS in Africa', *International Journal of STD and AIDS*, 14: 431–6.

Buve, A., Bishikwabo-Nsarhaza, K. and Mutangadura, G. (2002) 'The spread and effect of HIV-1 infection in sub-Saharan Africa', *The Lancet*, 359: 2011–17.

Cáceres, C.F., Marin, B.V. and Hudes, E.S. (2000) 'Sexual coercion among youth and young adults in Lima, Peru', *Journal of Adolescent Health*, 27: 361–7.

Caldwell, J.C., Caldwell, P., Caldwell, B.K. and Pieris, I. (1998) 'The construction of adolescence in a changing world: Implications for sexuality, reproduction, and marriage', *Studies in Family Planning*, 29: 137–53.

Centers for Disease Control and Prevention (CDC) (2003) *YRBSS Youth Outline: Comprehensive Results*. Online. Available HTTP: <http://apps.nccd.cdc.gov/yrbss/> (accessed 18 July 2005).

Coker, A.L., Richter, D.L., Valois, R.F., McKeown, R.E., Garrison, C.Z. and Vincent, M.L. (1994) 'Correlates and consequences of early initiation of sexual intercourse', *Journal of School Health*, 64: 372–7.

Cooksey, E.C., Mott, F.L. and Neubauer, S.A. (2002) 'Friendships and early relationships: Links to sexual initiation among American adolescents born to young mothers', *Perspectives on Sexual and Reproductive Health*, 34: 118–26.

Darroch, J.E. and Singh, S. (1999) *Why is Teenage Pregnancy Declining? The Roles of Abstinence, Sexual Activity and Contraceptive Use. Occasional Report No. 1*, New York: Alan Guttmacher Institute.

Darroch, J.E., Singh, S. and Frost, J.J. (2001) 'Differences in teenage pregnancy rates among five developed countries: The roles of sexual activity and contraceptive use', *Family Planning Perspectives*, 33: 244–50 and 281.

Dehne, K.L. and Riedner, G. (2001) 'Adolescence: A dynamic concept', *Reproductive Health Matters*, 9: 11–15.

Dickson, N., Paul, C., Herbison, P. and Silva, P. (1998) 'First sexual intercourse: Age, coercion, and later regrets reported by a birth cohort', *British Medical Journal*, 316: 29–33.

Dilley, J.W., Woods, W.J. and McFarlane, W. (1997) 'Are advances in treatment changing views about high-risk sex?' *New England Journal of Medicine*, 337: 501–2.

Dowsett, G., Aggleton, P., Abega, S.C., Jenkins, C., Marshall, T.M., Runganga, A., Schifter, J., Tan, M.L. and Tarr, C.M. (1998) 'Changing gender relations among young people: The global challenge for HIV/AIDS prevention', *Critical Public Health*, 8: 291–310.

Edgardh, K. (2002) 'Sexual behaviour in a low-income high school setting in Stockholm', *International Journal of STD and AIDS*, 13: 160–7.

Furstenberg, F. (1998) 'When will teenage childbearing become a problem? The implications of western experience for developing countries', *Studies in Family Planning*, 29: 246–53.

Futterman, D. (2003) *Youth and HIV: The Epidemic Continues*. Summary by Tim Horn. Online. Available HTTP: <http://www.prn._nb_cntnt/vol8/num1/flutter man_sum.htm> (accessed 27 November 2003).

Garofalo, R., Wolf, R.C., Kessel, S., Palfrey, J. and Durant, R.H. (1998) 'The association between health risk behaviors and sexual orientation among a school-based sample of adolescents', *Pediatrics*, 101: 895–902.

Grulich, A.E., de Visser, R.O., Smith, A.M.A., Rissel, C.E. and Richters, J. (2003) 'Sex in Australia: Homosexual experience and recent homosexual encounters', *Australian and New Zealand Journal of Public Health*, 27: 155–63.

Grunbaum, J., Kann, L., Kinchen, S.A., Williams, B., Ross, J.G., Lowry, G. and Kolbe, L. (2002) 'Youth risk behavior surveillance: United States, 2001', in *Surveillance Summaries, June 2002, MMWR 2002: 51 (No. SS-4)*, Atlanta: Centers for Disease Control and Prevention, pp. 1–21.

Gupta, G.R. (2003) 'Lessons from the past, challenges for the future: An overview of HIV/AIDS in Africa.' Plenary presentation *HIV/AIDS in Africa: What works*. Center for Global Development and John Snow Inc., 8 January 2003, Washington, DC. Online. Available HTTP: <http://www.icrw.org/docs/grg_speech_csis_022603.doc> (accessed 1 November 2004).

Irvine, J.M. (1994) *Sexual Cultures and the Construction of Adolescent Identities*. Health, Society, and Policy series, Philadelphia: Temple University Press.

Jackson, P. (2001) 'Pre-gay, post-queer: Thai perspectives on proliferating gender/sex diversity in Asia', *Journal of Homosexuality*, 40: 1–26.

Jessor, S.L. and Jessor, R. (1977) *Problem Behavior and Psychosocial Development: A Longitudinal Study of Youth*, New York: Academic Press.

Keys, D. (2003) 'Non-heterosexual young women in the Project i Study.' Conference presentation, *Towards Informed Practice: Lesbian Health Research at ARCSHS*, Melbourne: Australian Research Centre in Sex, Health and Society, La Trobe University. Details of Project i can be obtained from: http://www.kcwh.unimelb.edu.au/projecti/

Kirby, D. (2001) *Emerging Answers: Research Findings on Programs to Reduce Teen Pregnancy*, Washington, DC: National Campaign to Prevent Teen Pregnancy.

Kirby, D. (2002) *Do Abstinence-only Programs Delay the Initiation of Sex Among Young People and Reduce Teen Pregnancy?*, Washington, DC: National Campaign to Prevent Teen Pregnancy.

Larimer, M., Lydum, A., Anderson, B. and Turner, A. (1999) 'Male and female recipients of unwanted sexual contact in a college student sample: Prevalence rates, alcohol use, and depression symptoms', *Sex Roles: A Journal of Research*, 40: 295–308.

Luke, N. and Kurz, K.M. (2002) *Cross-generational and Transactional Sexual Relations in Sub-Saharan Africa* (ICRW, PSI). Online. Available HHTP: <http://www.icrw.org/docs/CrossGenSex_Report_902.pdf> (accessed 2 November 2004).

Mallett, S., Edwards, J., Keys, D., Myers, P. and Rosenthal, D. (2003) *Disrupting Stereotypes: Young People, Drug Use and Homelessness*, Melbourne: The Key Centre in Women's Health in Society, University of Melbourne.

Moore, S. and Rosenthal, D. (1993) *Sexuality in Adolescence*. Adolescence and Society series, London and New York: Routledge.

O'Donnell, L., O'Donnell, C.R. and Stueve, A. (2001) 'Early sexual initiation and subsequent sex-related risks among urban minority youth: The Reach for Health Study', *Family Planning Perspectives*, 33: 268–75.

Panchaud, C., Singh, S., Feivelson, D. and Darrogh, J.E. (2000) 'Sexually transmitted diseases among adolescents in developed countries', *Family Planning Perspectives*, 32: 24–32 and 45.

Panos Institute (2001) *Young Men and HIV: Culture, Poverty and Sexual Risk*, Geneva/London: UNAIDS/The Panos Institute. Online. Available HTTP: <http://www.panos.org.uk/PDF/reports/youngmenandhivculture.pdf> (accessed 2 November 2004).

Population Information Program (2001) *Youth and HIV/AIDS: Can we avoid catastrophe?* Series L, Number 12, 29(3), Maryland, USA: Center for Communication Programs, The Johns Hopkins University, Bloomberg School of Public Health.

Population Reference Bureau (2001) *Youth in Sub-Saharan Africa: A Chartbook of Sexual Experience and Reproductive Health*. Online. Available HTTP: <http://222.phishare.org/files/107_YouthSubSaharanAfrica.pdf> (accessed 2 November 2004).

Remez, L. (2000) 'Oral sex among adolescents: Is it sex or is it abstinence?' *Family Planning Perspectives*, 32: 298–305.

Reynolds, R. (2002) *From Camp to Queer*, Melbourne, Australia: Melbourne University Press.

Rissel, C.E., Richters, J., Grulich, A.E., de Visser, R.O. and Smith, A.M.A. (2003) 'First experiences of vaginal intercourse and oral sex among a representative sample of adults', *Australian and New Zealand Journal of Health*, 27: 131–7.

Rosario, M., Meyer-Bahlburg, H.F., Hunter, J. and Gwadz, M. (1999) 'Sexual risk behaviors of gay, lesbian, and bisexual youths in New York City: Prevalence and correlates', *AIDS Education and Prevention*, 11: 476–96.

Rosenthal, D. (1997) 'Understanding sexual coercion among young adolescents: Communicative clarity, pressure, and acceptance', *Archives of Sexual Behaviour*, 26: 481–93.

Rosenthal, D., Moore, S. and Buzwell, S. (1994) 'Homeless youths: Sexual and drug-related behaviour, sexual beliefs and HIV/AIDS risk', *AIDS Care*, 6: 83–94.

Rosenthal, D. and Smith, A.M.A. (1997) 'Adolescent sexual timetables', *Journal of Youth and Adolescence*, 26: 619–36.

Rosenthal, D., Smith, A.M.A. and de Visser, R.O. (1999) 'Personal and social factors influencing age at first intercourse', *Archives of Sexual Behavior*, 28: 319–33.

Rosenthal, S.L., Von Ranson, K.M., Cotton, S., Biro, F.M., Mills, L. and Succop, P.A. (2001) 'Sexual initiation: Predictors and developmental trends', *Sexually Transmitted Diseases*, 28: 527–32.

Shanler, S., Heise, L., Stewart, L. and Weiss, E. (1998) *Sexual Abuse and Young Adult Reproductive Health, In Focus: Focus on Young Adults*, Watertown, WA: Pathfinder International. Online. Available HTTP: <http://www.pathfind.org/pf/pubs/focus/IN%20FOCUS/sexabuseinfocus.html> (accessed 2 November 2004).

Silberschmidt, M. and Rasch, V. (2001) 'Adolescent girls, illegal abortions and 'sugar-daddies' in Dar es Salaam: Vulnerable victims and active social agents', *Social Science and Medicine*, 52: 1815–26.

Singh, S., Wulf, D., Samara, R. and Cuca, Y.P. (2000) 'Gender differences in the timing of first intercourse: Data from 14 countries', *International Family Planning Perspectives*, 26: 21–8 and 43.

Smith, A.M.A., Agius, P., Dyson, S., Mitchell, A. and Pitts, M. (2003) *Secondary Students and Sexual Health 2002*, Melbourne: Australian Research Centre in Sex, Health and Society, La Trobe University.

Stanton, B., Li, X., Black, M.M., Ricardo, I. and Galbraith, J. (1994) 'Anal intercourse among preadolescent and early adolescent low-income urban African-Americans', *Archives of Pediatrics and Adolescent Medicine*, 148: 1201–4.

Strathdee, S.A., Martindale, S.L., Cornelisse, P.G.A., Miller, M., Craib, J.P., O'Shaunessy, M.V. and Hogg, R.S. (2000) 'HIV infection and risk behaviours among young gay and bisexual men in Vancouver', *Canadian Medical Association Journal*, 162: 21–5.

Tai-hwan, K., Hee, J.K. and Sung-nam, C. (1999) 'Sexuality, contraception and abortion among unmarried adolescents and young adults: The case of Korea', in A.I. Mundigo and C. Indriso (eds) *Abortion in the Developing World*, New Delhi: Vistaar Publications and WHO, pp. 346–67.

Tan, M. (2001) 'Survival through pluralism: Emerging gay communities in the Philippines', *Journal of Homosexuality*, 40, 117–42.

UNAIDS (1999) *Sex and Youth: Contextual Factors Affecting Risk for HIV/AIDS: A Comparative Analysis of Multi-site Studies in Developing Countries*, Geneva: UNAIDS.

UNAIDS (2000) *Report on the Global HIV/AIDS Epidemic*, Geneva: UNAIDS.

UNAIDS (2002) *Report on the Global HIV/AIDS Epidemic*, Geneva: UNAIDS.

UNAIDS/WHO (2002) *AIDS Epidemic Update*, Geneva: UNAIDS/WHO.

UNFPA (2003) *State of World Population*, New York: UNFPA.

UNICEF (2001) *A League Table of Teenage Births in Rich Nations*, New York: UNICEF.

UNICEF, UNAIDS and WHO (2002) *Young People and HIV/AIDS: Opportunity in Crisis*, New York and Geneva: UNICEF/UNAIDS/WHO.

Van Landingham, M. (2002) 'Recent changes in heterosexual attitudes, norms and behaviors among unmarried Thai men: a qualitative analysis', *International Family Planning Perspectives*, 28: 6–15.

Waldo, C.R., McFarland, W., Katz, M.H., MacKellar, D. and Valleroy, L.A. (2000) 'Very young gay and bisexual men are at risk for HIV infection: The San Francisco Bay Area young men's survey II', *Journal of Acquired Immune Deficiency Syndromes*, 24: 168–74.

Weiss, E., Whelan, D. and Gupta, G.R. (2000) 'Gender, sexuality and HIV: Making a difference in the lives of young women in developing countries', *Sexual and Relationship Therapy*, 15: 233–45.

Wellings, K., Nanchahal, K., Macdowall, W., McManus, S., Erens, B., Mercer, C.H., Johnson, A.M., Copas, A.J., Korovessis, C., Fenton, K.A. and Field, J. (2001) 'Sexual behaviour in Britain: Early heterosexual experience', *The Lancet*, 358: 1843–50.

Youn, G. (2001) 'Perceptions of peer sexual activities in Korean adolescents', *Journal of Sex Research*, 38: 352–60.

Zavodny, M. (2001) 'The effect of partners' characteristics on teenage pregnancy and its resolution', *Family Planning Perspectives*, 33: 192–9 and 205.

Chapter 6

Young people and illicit drug use

Neil Hunt

All over the world, concern has been expressed about young people's use of illicit drugs such as cannabis, inhalants, tranquillisers, amphetamine-type stimulants, cocaine and heroin. Social surveys consistently identify drug use as a widespread activity among young people. Usually, it occurs within a variably sized minority of the youthful population. More rarely, surveys find that lifetime drug use is reported by a majority of young people (Ramsay *et al.* 2001, Johnston *et al.* 2004). Studies of certain groups of young people such as young offenders, children excluded from school, children in care or regular club-goers commonly find that in these contexts drug use is statistically the norm, rather than the exception (Green *et al.* 2000; Hamilton *et al.* 2000; Melrose and Brodie 2000; Winstock, Griffiths and Stewart 2001).

The most widely available data measure prevalence, or the proportion of the population using drugs within a given period. Data are usually collected by self-report, that is by asking people whether and what drugs they have used. Measures of the prevalence of drug use are greatly affected by the time period under scrutiny. The most inclusive measure, yielding the highest prevalence rates, comes from lifetime drug use. While this can be a useful indicator of exposure to drug use during development, and is of sociological interest as a marker of drug use within society, it has many limitations as a measure that relates in any way to problems or need. Lifetime measures include drug use that may have occurred years earlier and relate poorly to current consumption patterns. They say almost nothing about the nature of the use and the extent to which it might be problematic or remain in any way relevant, within the person's life.

Measures of use in the past year or month offer more sensitive indicators and thus offer a more helpful guide to current drug use. However, if there is no detail of the extent and nature of use these also have marked limitations. Taking a single smoke on a cannabis joint and smoking several grams of cannabis daily would be indistinguishable as responses to a dichotomous yes/no question about use in the past year. For these reasons, an understanding of drug-type, frequency and amount of use, and mode of administration are all desirable and important refinements to the information needed for a proper understanding of young people's drug use. With these issues and limitations in mind, it is useful to look at some international comparisons in reported patterns of use.

The Americas

Within the USA, the National Institute on Drug Abuse (NIDA) has funded a school-based survey – *Monitoring the Future* – since 1975. This currently gathers data on young people at ages 13–14, 15–16 and 17–18 (Johnston *et al.* 2004). Findings reveal trends that tend to be replicated in similar studies, and will be described in some detail before a more selective comparison of similarities and differences among young people elsewhere around the world. Other than where indicated, all comparisons come from a recent United Nations review of the world situation regarding youth drug use (United Nations 2001).

In 2003, 22.8 per cent of young people aged 13–14 in the USA reported having used an illicit drug during their lifetime, rising to 51.1 per cent of young people aged 17–18. Restricting our attention to the group with highest rates – twelfth graders – cannabis use explains much of the illicit use, constituting 46.1 per cent of lifetime use. However, for this age group, the more sensitive measures of cannabis use in the past thirty days and daily use are lower, at 21.2 per cent and 6 per cent respectively. Daily use is a more useful indicator of problematic use and it is noteworthy that this occurs at a much lower rate than lifetime or recent use – a trend that is sustained across all substances.

Importantly, lifetime use of alcohol (76.6 per cent) and cigarettes (53.7 per cent) exceeds that for cannabis, as does daily use of tobacco (8.4 per cent). However, daily use of alcohol is less common (3.2 per cent).

In contrast, lifetime use of heroin (1.5 per cent), cocaine powder (7.7 per cent) and crack cocaine (3.6 per cent) is reported more rarely, with recent use only reported by a very small minority of 17–18 year olds. This is suggestive of judicious discrimination between the risks of different substances and is consistent with other evidence concerning the way in which risks are differentially perceived by young people in a way that largely reflects the hazards they generate. Intermediate lifetime use rates are reported for other substances such as hallucinogens (10.6 per cent), tranquillisers (10.2 per cent) and MDMA/ecstasy (8.3 per cent). The ready availability of inhalants/volatile substances may explain why their use occurs at relatively high levels (11.2 per cent) in relation to the serious hazards they present.

In Canada, studies such as the Ontario Students Drug Survey and the Nova Scotia Students Drug Use Survey reveal very similar patterns to those in the USA, with lifetime prevalence declining from higher levels of lifetime use for cannabis and then hallucinogens, down through amphetamines and cocaine towards low rates of opiate use.

Central American countries tend to report a lower prevalence of lifetime use. A study of 12–18 year olds in Guatemala found that the lifetime prevalence of cannabis use was only 3 per cent, although there was evidence that the use of inhalants was more common. By contrast, in Panama, tranquillisers appear more popular, with up to 7 per cent of young people having tried them. In Mexico, against a background of increasing adult drug use during the 1990s, a household survey of 12–17 year olds in 1998 found cannabis use within the past twelve months reported by 2.4 per cent of males and 0.45 per cent of females with approximately half these numbers reporting the use of inhalants or cocaine (Medina-Mora and Rojas 2003; Medina-Mora *et al.* 2003).

The Caribbean has little data on youth substance use although there is evidence from the early 1990s of lifetime cannabis use by about 17 per cent of young people in Jamaica and Barbados. However, this was reported by only 1.8 per cent of young people in the Dominican Republic. Cocaine use is believed to be growing across the region.

Cannabis is, again, the main drug that is reported by young people across South America. Although lifetime use is generally tending to increase across the continent, rates are substantially lower than within Europe or North America and there is considerable variation between countries. Thus, lifetime cannabis use is reported to be low, at 1.8 per cent, among 17–19 year olds in Peru and also within a Venezuelan school survey. The rate increases in Bolivia – 3.5 per cent of 12 to 21 year olds; Uruguay – 3.7 per cent of 12–19 year olds; Ecuador students – 3.9 per cent; Brazil – 7.6 per cent of 10–18 year olds; Colombia – 9.2 per cent of 12–24 year olds and Chile – 11.1 per cent of 12 to 18 year olds. Tranquillisers, hallucinogens and inhalants are used at lower rates and, consistent with its production in several countries across the region, rates of cocaine and coca paste are often second to those for cannabis. Within Brazil, the lifetime cannabis rate reflects a rising trend that has increased threefold among 10–18 year olds between 1987 (2.8 per cent) and 1997 (7.9 per cent) (Galduroz *et al.* 2004). Although rare, some indications of heroin use have recently been noted across the region.

Africa

Data quality in Africa frequently limits what can be said about patterns of drug use among young people in many countries. In general, reported rates appear to be lower than in most industrialised countries, yet with signs that they are tending to increase. Other than alcohol and tobacco, lifetime use of inhalants appears more common than any other drug including cannabis: Kenya (19 per cent), Swaziland (12 per cent) and Zimbabwe (12 per cent). Cannabis use nevertheless appears to be common, alongside low rates of heroin and cocaine use. There is some evidence that rates of heroin use are growing in countries including the United Republic of Tanzania and

South Africa. There are also some important regional differences, with more widespread use of the stimulant *khat* in eastern Africa and the depressant methaqualone in parts of South Africa such as Cape Town. More recently, within a sample of 2,732 Cape Town 15–16 year olds derived from a school survey, Parry *et al.* (2004) have reported lifetime use of: cannabis 32 per cent (males) and 13.1 per cent (females); Mandrax 5.7 per cent (males) and 1.9 per cent (females); inhalants 15.8 per cent (males) and 4.9 per cent (females); ecstasy 4.3 per cent (males) and 3.1 per cent (females) and crack cocaine 2.6 per cent (males) and 1.0 per cent (females).

Asia

Despite limitations on the quality and comparability of Asian data, in many countries, amphetamines are among the more widely used drugs. Prior to a severe crackdown in Thailand, 5.6 per cent of Thai youth reported having used methamphetamines, which are also reported in the Philippines (4.3 per cent) Vientiane, Laos (4.8 per cent) and Japan (0.5 per cent). Lifetime use of any drug was reported by 28 per cent of students in Cambodia during 1997. Although China's cannabis consumption appears to be low, more than half of her heroin users are aged under 25 and ecstasy use appears to be growing. Problems associated with injecting and HIV/AIDS are rapidly growing within China.

In Nepal, 1992 data suggested that lifetime use of heroin (2.5 per cent) was a little under half the rate for cannabis (6.1 per cent), whereas in part of southern India cannabis had been used by 27 per cent of students. In this same context, recent increases in opiate injecting and HIV/AIDS have come to dominate public health concerns. Injecting is also a particular concern in central Asia within countries associated with heroin production or that are transit points in its distribution, such as Afghanistan, Pakistan, Kyrgyzstan and Iran. Again, heroin use sometimes exceeds the use of cannabis, as in Tashkent, Uzbekistan where among 25.9 per cent of drug users 78.5 per cent had used heroin but only 14 per cent reported cannabis use.

Europe

The European Monitoring Centre on Drugs and Drug Addiction (EMCDDA) collates data from EU states and produces an annual report that allows inter-country comparisons to be made (EMCDDA 2003a). In relative terms, many of the same general patterns are evident within EU data. However, there is considerable variation in absolute levels of substance use. So, regarding cannabis for example, among 15–16 year olds, lifetime prevalence ranges from countries with low rates as in Portugal (8 per cent), Sweden (8 per cent), Greece (9 per cent), and Finland (10 per cent) to others with relatively high rates: Spain (30 per cent), Ireland (32 per cent), France (35 per cent) and the

UK (35 per cent). Whereas there is a preponderance of problematic use among males within the adult population, lifetime prevalence of illicit drugs tends to be more similar among school-age males and females. Some gender variations are nevertheless observed, such as the greater prevalence of use of tranquillisers and non-prescribed sedatives among girls.

The EMCDDA also collates data from states that have recently joined the EU and other candidate countries (Bulgaria, Romania and Turkey) (EMCDDA 2003b). Lifetime use of any drug among 16 year olds varies from 12 per cent in Romania to 35 per cent in the Czech Republic, with cannabis making the most substantial contribution to these data. A notable exception is Romania where only 1 per cent of young people report having tried cannabis but 8 per cent have tried heroin. As elsewhere, alcohol looms largest, with over 90 per cent of 16 year olds having tried it and nearly two thirds having been drunk on one or more occasions.

Indeed, heroin use is generally more common in East rather than West Europe (for example within Latvia, Lithuania and Croatia) and there are particular concerns within the Russia Federation, which has the highest levels of heroin injecting among 15–16 year olds – with corresponding concerns regarding HIV/AIDS spread (UNODCCP 2002).

Oceania

Patterns of substance use among young people in Australia and New Zealand share many similarities with those in North America, with the lifetime prevalence of illicit drugs being highest for cannabis and lowest for heroin. Perhaps because of the region's growing economic and cultural ties with south-eastern Asia, however, it seems that methamphetamine base or the smokeable 'ice' or 'pure' is now becoming more common.

Patterns of use

The data so far described offer a somewhat crude insight into young people's patterns of drug use. They need to be supplemented by other information if we are to more fully understand young people's relationships to drugs. In particular, important distinctions need to be made between young people trying drugs largely out of curiosity, young people routinely using them instrumentally as part of their leisure lifestyle and young people whose use of drugs has come substantially to dominate their focus and activities within life. It is commonplace to discuss patterns of drug use in terms that reflect these broad distinctions – i.e. with reference to experimental, recreational and problematic/dependent use.

As its name suggests, *experimental use* is largely concerned with the formative testing out of the effects of a drug, typically driven in considerable part by curiosity. Either through direct social exposure or the media, a range of drugs are part of the social landscape for most young people and experimentation is one important way by which many young people seek to learn about their effects and gain a better understanding of these substances, which are simultaneously vilified and lionised by different members of their society. Just as many people might ride a large amusement park ride to see what it is like and, perhaps, to be able to tell others that they have done so – experimental drug use fulfils a somewhat similar function. Doing so does not necessarily signal a desire to spend every weekend on a ten loop ride that generates a G-force of 3.5, merely the desire to know what it is like to do it once which, for many people, is as many times as they will ever want to do it.

Recreational use, on the other hand, refers to drug-taking that happens more instrumentally yet mostly without immediate problems. Most often this denotes drug-taking such as the use of cannabis for relaxation and socialisation, or the periodic use of some combination of ecstasy, amphetamines or hallucinogens, often alongside alcohol and tobacco. Although drugs such as the ones mentioned are most widely used recreationally, it is the pattern of use that is defining, rather than the drugs themselves; so, contrary to the way these things are commonly conceived, some people might use heroin or crack cocaine 'recreationally' and drugs that are often considered relatively benign, such as cannabis, can result in a problematic or dependent pattern of use.

Problematic/dependent use, or addiction as many lay people think of it, is the pattern that generates the most concern, sometimes necessitating treatment. Physical or psychological dependence characterised by increasing tolerance, craving and a withdrawal syndrome contributes to a wider range of problems affecting mental and physical health, relationships, educational attainment or work and including legal problems associated with the criminalised status of drug possession or use. Many young people find the terms 'addict' 'drug misuser' or 'drug abuser' highly alienating, especially when they perceive these to be applied to themselves inaccurately – an important point to remember in any work that aims to engage young people effectively. Nevertheless, technically, there are two main sources of clinical definition that are widely used: 'dependence syndrome' from the International Classification of Diseases and Health Problems (World Health Organization 1992) and 'substance use and dependence' defined by the American Psychiatric Association in their *Diagnostic and Statistical Manual of Mental Disorders* (1994).

Although it does not occur so commonly in typologies of use, there is a strong argument for including *functional use* as something that is not necessarily problematic and is separate and distinct from recreational use, in that it is not use for leisure but is more concerned with performance/coping. It often relates to young people in difficult circumstances such as street children/youth or those in harsh economic situations. Examples include the use of stimulants to keep awake while working long hours or hypnosedatives to deal with stress, anxiety, depression and physical/sexual abuse (Ball and Howard 1995).

Etiology and causation

Given the immense stigma attached to young people's drug use, asking 'What did we do wrong?' is often the first reaction for parents or carers who discover that a child or young person is using drugs. High quality studies examining the relationship between parenting, psychological adjustment and substance use are rare within the literature. Typically, studies employ cross-sectional designs that take a single set of measures of different variables and then look for associations between these. However, 'one-shot', cross-sectional studies are poor at answering crucial questions about causality and long-term effects. To properly unpick these relationships, designs that follow people up over time are preferable, although their greater expense means that they are uncommon. One rare exception, published by Shedler and Block (1990), usefully aids our understanding of the family and psychological factors that predict experimentation and problematic substance use. Although it should be borne in mind that this study was conducted within the USA and may not be generalisable, it was a longitudinal investigation, undertaken with unusual rigour, which followed children from the age of 3 to 18 and gathered a series of measures of – among many other things – parenting quality, psychological adjustment and drug-taking.

In essence, 130 children were recruited into a study of ego and cognitive development at the age of 3. One hundred and one of these (49 boys, 52 girls) were successfully followed up with a battery of measures at the ages of 4, 5, 7, 11, 14, through to 18. At the age of 18, the participants were categorised as 'abstainers', 'experimenters' or 'frequent users' from several measures of substance use.

A large number of strong, statistically significant findings were noted. The experimenters emerged as the group that had both the best psychological adjustment and for whom maternal parenting quality was markedly better (paternal parenting was not significantly associated with outcomes): findings that were sustained from the earliest measurements taken, which means that they have important predictive value. In comparison to experimenters, the abstainers were 'relatively anxious, emotionally constricted and lacking in social skills'. Frequent users were judged to be relatively insecure, unable to form healthy relationships, and emotionally distressed at age 18 and rela-tively anxious, inhibited and morose as children. Compared with the mothers of experimenters, the mothers of both abstainers and frequent users were cold, critical, pressuring and unresponsive to their children's needs.

The importance of this study is that it suggests that early psychological adjustment may usefully assist the early identification of children and young people most at risk of developing problematic use and directs attention to aspects of parenting that protect children from frequent use. Such insights are of evident value for the development of programmes that aim to target interventions or support parents in developing ways of relating to their children that maximise their well-being and avert drug problems. It also offers corresponding reassurance to parents of experimenters who might ask 'What did we do wrong?' as the somewhat counter-intuitive conclusion is that, in terms of their parenting and their child's adjustment, things are more likely to have gone right.

The gateway theory

It is common to see references to the gateway theory in discussions about the development of problematic youth drug use (for example see the Runciman Report 2000). It is therefore important to consider the theory because it is widely referred to, yet also flawed. The theory proposes that the use of one drug leads to the use of other substances and the causation of drug problems. It is especially common for cannabis to be viewed in this way and such concerns contribute to calls for the preservation of serious controls on its availability (Golub and Johnson 2002). However, considerable care is needed because of the way the theory confuses a statistical artefact and causal processes.

It is undeniable that many people who are dependent on heroin, methamphetamine or cocaine will often have used cannabis: an observation that is frequently made within social and epidemiological research. However, only a small minority of cannabis users generally progress to using these other drugs, which suggests that, as a causal explanation, the gateway theory is weak (Golub and Johnson 2002).

To elaborate briefly, due to its widespread availability people with a general tendency to try drugs are more likely to encounter cannabis earlier and use it first. This is not the same as causation and many problematic users will have a range of other, more important risk factors that need to be taken into account (discussed later). Indeed, it is consistently found that the earlier and more extensive use of alcohol and tobacco is more prevalent among cannabis users, which means that – to the extent that any substance might be thought of as a gateway drug – it is tobacco or alcohol that might more meaningfully be understood in this way (Johnson *et al.* 2000).

Earlier and more extensive use of alcohol and tobacco is, nevertheless, associated with developing later, problematic use. Cannabis use is also associated with lower educational attainment (Johnson *et al.* 2000; Macleod *et al.* 2004a, 2004b). So, earlier and more extensive use can usefully be considered among the range of risk factors that may be helpful within programmes targeting people thought to have a heightened risk of developing problematic use. Nevertheless, as Macleod *et al.* (2004a, 2004b) are at pains to point out, such associations appear 'to be explicable in terms of non-causal mechanisms'. Consequently, these factors cannot reliably be viewed as predictive of any given person developing problems.

Peer preference not peer pressure

When asked why young people use drugs, adults and young people them-selves frequently give accounts that make reference to some form of peer pressure. This is probably one of the most commonly discussed risk factors for youth drug use. However, the available research shows that explanations in terms of peer pressure – in the sense of some external, imposed, coercive force – do not stand up to scrutiny to anything like the degree that this cause is invoked within explanations of youth drug use. Whilst the interplay in relationships between peers is, almost certainly, an important process, one of the most searching reviews of recent years, undertaken by Coggans and McKellar (1994), has shown that the literature on peer effects on drug-taking is frequently flawed, misinterpreted or over-interpreted.

Identified problems within the literature include: a lack of conceptual clarity and poor operationalisation of 'pressure' (e.g. interpreting 'tolerance of deviance' as 'susceptibility to pressure'), adopting 'pressure' explanations for data that can more parsimoniously be interpreted simply as preferring to mix with others who are similar, blurring 'peer support' with 'peer pressure', and drawing causal inferences from cross-sectional data that cannot readily sustain them. Simultaneously, studies that have produced negative findings with regard to peer pressure have been somewhat downplayed with an apparent reluctance to acknowledge the conclusions of studies that fly in the face of a peer pressure orthodoxy.

In contrast, there is much evidence showing that young people are more likely to seek like-minded peers who enable them to pursue activities they favour, including drug-taking. Such studies show the importance of being more attentive to the mechanisms by which young people find and select friends like themselves (peer assortment or homophily) and the way this relates to drug-taking. It seems that, in large part, young people largely seek out people like themselves, with whom they prefer to associate. They tend to do so because it is preferable to be with others who are similar and sup-portive of the activities they choose to participate in, especially where these are otherwise proscribed: leading to the conclusion that 'peer preference' gives a more powerful and plausible account of some of the widely observed relationships found within the research.

But how could such sustained and embedded problems in our under-standing of the role of peer pressure ever have arisen? Perhaps part of the explanation lies in the way that it may be convenient, and in many respects reassuring, for all parties to account for drug use in terms of peer pressure, regardless of its veracity. By doing so, adults can to some extent absolve young people of behaviour that remains largely stigmatised and demonised within society. Similarly, young people can partially displace responsibility for drug-taking from themselves to others. And of course, practitioners within drug education programmes that are based on peer pressure resistance also have a considerable interest in its continued existence. Together, these factors provide a collective, vested interest in denying the uncomfortable possibility that young people often choose to use drugs themselves because they sometimes find them enjoyable: a conclusion that pushes us to ask challenging questions about the proper emphasis of drug education programmes targeting young people and the expectations we might reasonably have of them.

Risk factors, protective factors and vulnerable groups

This chapter has already included some discussion of risk and protective factors, with reference to early psychological adjustment, parenting quality and early use of tobacco and alcohol. The better we understand the factors that put young people at risk of developing problems, and the more refined our appreciation of those that confer protection, the more wisely we can intervene through drug policy and any corresponding programmes.

Fortunately, a large number of risk and protective factors for problematic use are now more clearly recognised. Although much attention is quite rightly paid to intra-personal and inter-personal determinants, more recent literature on risk and protective factors increasingly forces a widening of our attention to include a focus on additional structural, economic, societal and cultural factors. This welcome shift has seen a burgeoning in our understanding of the potential targets for intervention – either as risk factors we might seek to minimise or protective factors we might promote – many of which are not directly concerned with drugs themselves, but underpin healthy development more generally.

Where risk factors cluster together the chances of problematic drug use occurring are magnified: further helping us identify those most at risk. It also seems that risk factors are generally more prevalent among certain groups of young people, such as young offenders, street children and the homeless, sex workers, children in care or children excluded from school. Although care is needed to avoid careless assumptions that membership of such groups denotes drug use, this insight nevertheless allows a more focused approach that can sensibly channel attention towards those young people where resources are more likely to be needed, rather than a diffuse approach that, less effectively, embraces all young people equally.

Because of the number and breadth of factors that are now recognised as relevant, it is not practical to discuss all of them in detail here. Instead, this section signposts and summarises some of the main conclusions from a few of the different points of reference that exist.

In the UK, the National Health Service Health Advisory Service's report 'Children and young people substance misuse services: the substance of young needs' (Health Advisory Service 1996) distinguishes between social and cultural risk factors such as substance availability and economic deprivation; individual and interpersonal risk factors such as parental substance use and family conflict; and protective factors such as the young person having a caring relationship with at least one adult.

This approach places attention on vulnerable groups within which drug-taking is more common and for whom risk factors are often aggregated. By doing so, it directs attention towards opportunities for effective, targeted programmes. So, for example, programmes focus on young offenders, young homeless, children within the care system, those who are excluded from school or who are regularly truanting, young people from minority ethnic groups within which certain substance use problems are concentrated, or young people who present with early problems associated with alcohol and tobacco. In each case, there are structural opportunities and points of contact within public services for the development of targeted programmes.

The assets approach within the USA places a particular emphasis on protective factors and details forty external and internal assets that promote healthy development (Benson *et al.* 2004). Among these, external assets are grouped in terms of support, empowerment, boundaries and expectations, and constructive use of time. Internal assets include: commitment to learning, positive values, social competencies, and positive identity.

In Australia, Spooner and colleagues (2001) have comprehensively reviewed the structural determinants of youth drug use. Although individual and interpersonal factors are of relevance for any understanding of youth drug use, their work is important because of the way it draws attention to the underpinning effects of deprivation and social capital – or its absence. Regarding deprivation, they highlight the impact of widening socio-economic differentials, low socio-economic status and their aggregated effects within particular communities to produce a risk environment. Within the social/cultural environment, Spooner *at al.* (2001) focus on social support and social cohesion and the way these are mediated by values and beliefs, changing leisure time, ethnic and workplace cultures and the media. They identify a range of ways in which these might be enhanced so that substance use problems might be reduced. In doing so, they also draw attention to the relevance of macro-economic policies regarding taxation, education and labour policy, which emerge as important components within any comprehensive programme that seriously engages with youth drug use. More particularly, Spooner *at al.* (2001) provide clear principles that would be expected to enhance drug prevention programmes. These include ensuring that programmes operate collaboratively with others addressing problem behaviours around crime, suicide and within education, and focusing programmes on developmental transitions.

A recent review of the evidence for preventing HIV/AIDS among young injecting drug users in Central and Eastern Europe/the Commonwealth of Independent States and the Baltics (Howard *et al.* 2003) draws attention to structural factors that may be of particular relevance to young people in countries with transitional and developing economies; notably increased social mobility, the break up of mechanisms of social control with their accompanying racial and religious tensions and the generalised effects of rapid economic change. The role of drug production and transit is also critical because of its impact on localised availability, for example with regard to amphetamine type stimulants in Asia, heroin transiting the Balkans or the impact of cocaine in parts of the Caribbean. Although economic and cultural factors sometimes mediate, with the result that production and transit do not relate directly to use; in general the two are closely linked. Often there are also corresponding interactions with the sex industry, the increasing use of young people for drug production, distribution and trafficking – as in some Brazilian *favelas* – and the near endemic use of drugs among street children.

Intervening intelligently in youth drug use

Primary prevention is concerned with preventing an illness, disease or adverse event from ever occurring. In relation to young people's substance use, primary prevention is mainly used to denote programmes that prevent young people from beginning drug-taking, i.e. averting drug experimentation. However, the recognition that early substance use is an important risk factor for problematic use means that delaying experimentation is, increasingly, a more realistic goal being adopted within primary prevention efforts.

The objective of secondary prevention efforts within youth substance use can best be regarded as the reduction of harm among those young people who use one or more substances, whether this might be experimentally or within a more regular pattern of recreational or dependent use. From a public health perspective it is, in a sense, immaterial whether a substance is used: the key concern is avoiding the harms that can result, although clearly if programmes can prevent substance use, this will most likely avert harm. The focus within secondary prevention is, therefore, on actions that can directly prevent harms among young drug users or, that avert an escalation of use towards levels that make problems such as dependence more likely. So, for example, environmental measures within clubs and dance parties to reduce the risk of heatstroke among ecstasy users or information that supports drug-using peer groups in setting and maintaining boundaries around their use of cocaine could both be classified as secondary prevention efforts. In recognition of the particular problems associated with injecting there is widespread recognition of the importance of needle and syringe programmes and also a growing interest in interventions that promote transitions from injecting or try to prevent people moving from, say, smoking heroin or sniffing amphetamine towards injecting (Hunt *et al.* 1999).

Tertiary prevention, on the other hand, is concerned with addressing the harms that have arisen in connection with use that has become problematic. In this respect, programmes for treating dependence or addressing other problems that can be associated with drug injecting, such as infection with HIV or hepatitis C, each constitute tertiary prevention.

Overwhelmingly, the largest area in which efforts to address youth drug use have taken place has been within school-based education. These commonly have primary prevention objectives. However, despite their widespread use the evidence suggests that they have very poor effectiveness. An extensive review for the World Health Organization (Hawks *et al.* 2002, x–xi) concludes that:

> While the majority of studies reviewed, deriving mainly from the United States, have abstinence as their goal, there is evidence that programmes having this goal consistently fail to produce behavioural effects suggesting that there is a need to develop programmes with outcomes other than abstinence as their goal.

Despite this pessimistic conclusion – one which forces us to ask hard questions of the nature and expectations of some of the programmes we implement – Hawks and his colleagues draw attention to several important points that have considerable salience in the light of the discussion throughout this chapter. They identify the importance of implementing programmes at a 'developmentally appropriate time . . . when interventions are most likely to have an impact on behaviour' (page 40). They also note that 'complementary general health/life skills programmes appear to produce greater change than skill-based education programmes alone' (page 41). And critically, they draw attention to the value of attending to risk and protective factors and drawing on a developing appreciation of the factors that produce young people who are resilient against problematic use despite the presence of multiple risk factors.

Beyond school-based programmes, a comprehensive approach needs to be directed towards those young people where risk factors are aggregated and where local or national epidemiology suggests drug use is more prevalent. In these vulnerable or at-risk groups, it is necessary for programmes to acknowledge that primary prevention is in most cases, largely, an unrealistic expectation and that drug use at levels well beyond those within the general population of young people will occur. In these circumstances, secondary prevention efforts need to incorporate intensive programmes to reduce risk factors and enhance protective factors alongside specific harm reduction efforts that are appropriate to the pattern and type of drug use that is likely to arise. For the most part, these will best be delivered in an integrated way within youth services, health and social care programmes and within the youth justice system.

In thinking through what works with regard to youth substance use, it is tempting to focus on programmes that directly address substance use itself. However, to exert the greatest effect and to truly engage with the most important factors that most contribute to problematic use, we must engage with underlying social conditions (Spooner *et al.* 2001). As long as young people's development occurs in circumstances characterised by relative economic deprivation and cultural impoverishment it is unrealistic to expect other programmes to perform a role that goes beyond a form of first aid.

Noteworthy exceptions to the rule that programmes need to be integrated with other youth services arise in connection with particular groups of young people. Two of these warrant particular mention: regular club-goers, where the clubbing environment and associated culture provides many valuable opportunities for targeted interventions and, crucially, young injecting drug users. Where there are populations of young injecting drug users, the provision of needle and syringe programmes that are adapted to their need are critical for the prevention of life-threatening infections including HIV/AIDS, hepatitis B and C; and life-saving interventions can be provided that aim both to prevent overdose and improve the way it is managed.

Finally, for the minority of young people who develop more serious problems there is a need for child- or youth-centred tertiary treatment services. In many respects, these need to parallel the range of services needed by adult drug users including work such as counselling, detoxification, substitution treatment, residential rehabilitation and crisis or respite services. However, in several important respects, there are differences.

The socio-legal context regarding confidentiality and the capacity to consent to treatment is typically different for young people to that within adult services. According to the age of the person, there may be a statutory requirement to involve the parents or carers and, in general, it will be highly desirable to do so. It is nevertheless important to take account of the feelings and views of the young person within this process – and indeed the treatment process as a whole. Where parents or carers have not been involved from the outset, it is usually preferable for this to be encouraged in a way where the young person is able to shape the terms on which this occurs. More rarely, as in cases where the parents or carers are contributing to the problems through an abusive relationship it will be inappropriate to involve them and it is sometimes necessary for a care plan to include measures that protect the young person from them.

The way in which young people's treatment is delivered must also be sensitive to their needs. Agreeing a suitable setting for treatment – not necessarily a specialist treatment service – and ensuring that services can respond flexibly with regard to the timing of contacts or appointments is essential. Services organised around the needs of practitioners, rather than the young person, are unlikely to engage and retain them.

The emphasis of the work is also likely to differ. Almost by definition, young people will have particular needs with regard to their general development and socialisation. This has an impact on the way in which their care addresses their educational or employment situation and the underpinning life skills necessary within the transition to independent living. Emotional issues are often prominent, in which problematic substance use can be inter-linked with formative relationship issues, especially where a partner also has problems with their own substance use: problems that are sometimes all the more complex where they or their partner are either pregnant or young parents.

Lastly, there is widespread recognition that young people usually benefit from services that are separate from those for older, adult substance users. There is a risk that services which mix young people within the same milieu as people with more entrenched problems can inadvertently worsen them. The optimum care pathway for someone who is at the early stage of a problem such as opioid dependence is not necessarily the same as that for someone whose use has extended over many years, and there are also evident risks of unintentionally widening the young person's social network in a way that enmeshes them with people whose problems are more entrenched.

References

American Psychiatric Association (1994) *Diagnostic and Statistical Manual of Mental Disorders, Fourth Edition*, Washington, DC: American Psychiatric Association.

Ball, A. and Howard, J. (1995) 'Psychoactive substance use among street children', in T. Harpham and I. Blue (eds) *Urbanization and Mental Health in Developing Countries*, Aldershot: Avebury.

Benson, P.L., Roehjkepartain, E.C. and Sesma, A. (2004) 'Tapping the power of community: building assets to strengthen substance abuse prevention', *Search Institute Insights and Evidence*, 2, 1: 1–14.

Coggans, N. and McKellar, S. (1994) 'Drug use amongst peers: peer pressure or peer preference?' *Drugs: Education, Prevention and Policy*, 1, 1: 15–26.

EMCDDA (2003a) *Annual report 2003: The state of the drugs problem in the European Union and Norway*, Lisbon: European Monitoring Centre on Drugs and Drug Addiction.

EMCDDA (2003b) *Annual report 2003: The state of the drugs problem in the acceding and candidate countries to the European Union*, Lisbon: European Monitoring Centre on Drugs and Drug Addiction.

Galduroz, J.C.F., Noto, A.R., Nappo, S.A. and Carlini, E.A (2004) 'Trends in drug use among students in Brazil: analysis of four surveys in 1987, 1989, 1993, and 1997', *Brazilian Journal of Medical and Biological Research*, 37: 523–31.

Golub, A. and Johnson, B.D. (2002) 'The misuse of the "Gateway Theory" in US policy on drug abuse control: A secondary analysis of the muddled deduction', *International Journal of Drug Policy*, 13: 5–19.

Green, C., Willoughby, R., Smith, A., Harris, P. and Crome, I. (2000) 'Determining drug use and evaluating effective assessment methods in a Youth Offending Team', in DrugScope, *Vulnerable young people and drugs: Opportunities to tackle inequalities*, London: DrugScope.

Hamilton, C., Sherwood, S., South, N., and Teeman, D. (2000) 'Drug interventions for looked after people', in DrugScope, *Vulnerable young people and drugs: Opportunities to tackle inequalities*, London: DrugScope.

Hawks, D., Scott, K., McBride, N., Jones, P. and Stockwell, T. (2002) *Prevention of psychoactive substance use: A selected review of what works in the area of prevention*, Geneva: World Health Organization.

Health Advisory Service (1996) *Children and young people substance misuse services: the substance of young needs*, London: HMSO.

Howard, J., Hunt, N. and Arcuri, A. (2003) *A situation assessment and review of the evidence for interventions for the prevention of HIV/AIDS among occasional, experimental and young injecting drug users*, background paper prepared for UN Interagency and CEEHRN Technical Consultation on Occasional, Experimental and Young IDUs in the CEE/CIS and Baltics.

Hunt, N., Griffiths, P., Southwell, M., Stillwell, G., and Strang, J. (1999) 'Preventing and curtailing injecting drug use: opportunities for developing and delivering "route transition interventions"', *Drug and Alcohol Review*, 18: 441–51.

Johnson, P.B., Boles, S.M. and Kleber, H.D. (2000) 'The relationship between adolescent smoking and drinking and likelihood estimates of illicit drug use', *Journal of Addictive Disease*, 19: 75–81.

Johnston, L.D., O'Malley, P.M., Bachman, J.G. and Schulenberg, J.E. (2004) *Monitoring the Future national survey results on drug use, 1975–2003. Volume I: Secondary school students* (NIH Publication No. 04-5507), Bethesda, MD: National Institute on Drug Abuse.

Macleod, J., Oakes, R., Copello, A., Crome, I., Egger, M., Hickman, M., Oppenkowski, T., Stokes-Lampard, H. and Davey Smith, G. (2004a) 'Psychological and social sequelae of cannabis and other illicit drug use by young people: a systematic review of longitudinal, general population studies', *The Lancet*, 363: 1579–88.

Macleod J., Oakes R., Oppenkowski T., Stokes-Lampard, H., Copello, A., Crome, I., Davey Smith, G., Egger, M., Hickman, M. and Judd, A. (2004b) 'How strong is the evidence that illicit drug use by young people is an important cause of psychological or social harm? Methodological and policy implications of a systematic review of longitudinal, general population studies', *Drugs: Education, Prevention and Policy*, 11: 281–97.

Medina-Mora, M.E. and Rojas, E. (2003) 'Demand for drugs: Mexico in the international perspective', *Salud Mental*, 26(2): 1–11.

Medina-Mora, M.E., Cravioto, P., Villatoro, J., Feliz, C., Galván-Castillo, F. and Tapia-Conyer, R. (2003) 'Drug use among adolescents: results from the National Survey of Addictions, 1998', *Salud Publica de Mexico*, 45: S16–S25 Suppl. 1.

Melrose, M. and Brodie, I. (2000) 'Vulnerable young people and their vulnerability to drug misuse', in DrugScope, *Vulnerable young people and drugs: Opportunities to tackle inequalities*, London: DrugScope.

Parry, C.D.H., Myers, B., Morojele, N.K., Flisher, A.J., Bhana, A., Donson, H. and Plüddemann, A. (2004) 'Trends in adolescent alcohol and other drug use: findings from three sentinel sites in South Africa (1997–2001)', *Journal of Adolescence*, 27: 429–40.

Ramsay, M., Baker, P., Goulden, C., Sharp, C. and Sondhi, A. (2001) *Drug Misuse declared in 2000: Results from the British Crime Survey*, Home Office Research Study 224, Home Office: London.

Runciman Report (2000) *Report of the independent inquiry into the Misuse of Drugs Act 1971*, London: The Police Foundation.

Shedler, J. and Block, J. (1990) 'Adolescent drug use and psychological health: a longitudinal inquiry', *American Psychologist*, 45, 5: 612–30.

Spooner, C., Hall, W. and Lynskey, M. (2001) *Structural determinants of youth drug use*, ANCD research paper 2. Woden ACT: Australian National Council on Drugs.

United Nations (2001) *World situation with regard to drug abuse, with particular reference to children and youth*, Economic and Social Council: E/CN.7/2001/4.

UNODCCP (2002) *Global illicit drug trend*, New York: United Nations Office for Drug Control and Crime Prevention.

Winstock, A.R., Griffiths, P. and Stewart, D. (2001) 'Drugs and the dance music scene: a survey of current drug use patterns among a sample of dance music enthusiasts in the UK', *Drug and Alcohol Dependence*, 64, 1: 9–17.

World Health Organization (1992) *The ICD-10 classification of mental and behavioural disorders: Clinical descriptions and diagnostic guidelines, tenth revision*, Geneva: World Health Organization.

Chapter 7

Drug use among same-sex attracted young people

John Howard and Anthony Arcuri

> In the car the other day, a group of us heading toward the beach, The Verve's The Drugs Don't Work came on the radio. A friend yelled out 'Get better drugs'. We all laughed, but my laughter was half hearted. The drugs don't work anymore, not like they used to. . . . People around me, they need drugs to love. That disturbs me. What if the drugs really didn't work? What then? No dance parties, no clubs no scene, no Mardi Gras? No queer, no gay?
>
> (Chris Tsiolkas, author of *Loaded*, cited in Murnane *et al.* 2000: 11)

Substance use, sexuality and sexual behaviour intersect on a number of levels, and substances have a variety of meanings for young people. Private and public consumption, and the context of, and reasons for, use can vary considerably.

For example, substances can be used to ease social situations such as parties in which sexual activity is anticipated or desired, to enhance sexual 'pleasure' (for example, the use of cocaine, amyl nitrite), to induce or maintain an erection and/or delay ejaculation (for example, the use of Viagra), or to render a potential sexual partner available by making them intoxicated. Intoxication can also be used as an excuse for inadequate sexual performance, or to excuse desired unsafe sexual activity such as the avoidance of condom use and/or violent and abusive sex.

Among young sex workers, substances such as benzodiazepines can be used to dull the pain of sexual activity, be payment for sex, render individuals less likely to refuse sex, get them sexually aroused, increase pleasure for the client, encourage certain sexual acts, facilitate involvement in the production of pornography, or decrease the chance that the young person could identify customers later. Also, substances can be used to induce intoxication in clients so as to avoid prolonged sexual activity and, later, to help the young person to forget that they have been involved in sex work. Drugs can also be used to reduce pain or as muscle relaxants to enable penetrative sex.

Substances can also be used to try to induce a termination of pregnancy and to ease transitions between public and private sexual identities or behaviour; for example, apparently heterosexual men having sex with other men, or moving from more normative patterns of sexual activity to more exotic or bizarre behaviour. Substance use also has a role to play in celebrations related to sexuality, such as 'coming out' in some same-sex attracted subcultures.

Most of the above associations between sexuality and substance use can apply to young people of whatever sexual orientation. However, this chapter will focus on the role of substance use in identity formation and sexual behaviour of same-sex attracted (SSA) young people: be they 'out', 'coming out' or 'confused' about their sexual identity.

It is imperative to note that while the term same-sex attracted is intended to be inclusive of many expressions of sexuality, sexual behaviour and identity, the term and others such as 'out' and 'coming out' pertain mostly to Western notions of sexuality and sexual behaviour. In the Western dominated literature and discourse, *men who have sex with men* is a term in common usage and has been intended to cover all males who have sex with other males. In other cultures and contexts, this term is more problematic (Khan 1999). As Gosine and Binswanger (2004: 9) suggest: 'Ideas about sex and sexuality are not universal. In low-income countries few people who have sexual relationships with members of the same gender necessarily identify as lesbian or gay'. They also note that recent research indicates that the terms *gay men* and *men who have sex with men* are not interchangeable, and point to the fluidity of male and female sexual experience (Davies *et al.* 1993). The term *male to male* has been preferred by writers such as Bondyopadhyay and Kahn (2004), as much sexual behaviour occurs where the penetrated person does not perceive himself as a man, but the penetrator does not perceive himself as anything but a man. This understanding applies in South Asia, the Middle East, Africa, the machismo cultures of Latin America, within immigrant groups and probably more broadly in Western countries.

Examples of diversity abound, and it is recognized that war, poverty, incarceration and institutional living arrangements such as migrant work camps, boarding schools, military establishments and seminaries result in single sex enclaves in which non-gay identified men have sex with men. While *gay* and *lesbian* are emerging labels within developing countries, there is no shortage of terms to describe same-sex sexual activity and identity. For example, among males the following terms may be used:

- *Azande* (men who buy boys to act as their wives) in the Central African Republic.
- *Ibbi* (men with feminine characteristics) in Senegal.
- *Sbikiro* (men blessed with the female spirit) in Zimbabwe.
- *Yan daudu* (men who dress as women) in Nigeria.
- *Hijra* (men of religious and cultural significance who sacrifice their genitalia and act as women), *kothi* (self-identified feminized males),

panthi (men who take an active role in penetration), *da-paratha* (males who penetrate and who are penetrated) in India.
- *Kathoey* (feminized men and transgendered persons) in Thailand.
- *Bakla* (feminized men and transgendered persons) in the Philippines.
- *Boroh pith brakat* (masculine men), *kteuy* (men who dress and act as women), *pros saat* (handsome, 'short hair' men and heterosexual men who have sex with other males), *pros luk kluan* (taxi boys who sell sex), *sak veng* (long hair, transgender men), *sray sros* (charming girls, transgender) in Cambodia.
- *Bugarrón* (penetrator), *pájaro* (the penetrated) and *maricón* ('fag'), *berdache* (two-spirited person) in the Dominican Republic.
- *Loca* (queen), *cacheros* (heterosexual men who have sex with men, often for money) in Costa Rica.

(Aggleton 1999, Gosine and Binswanger 2004, KHANA and the International HIV/AIDS Alliance 2003)

Likewise, there is major diversity in the spaces within which male to male sex occurs. These spaces may include brothels, open public spaces such as parks, toilets in shopping centres, bars and universities, in cars, sex clubs and homes. Much of this sexual activity can be furtive and quick, and, at times, with virtually no verbal communication. Gay discos are present or emerging in some developing and transitional countries, but in others meeting places remain limited and hidden.

In what follows, there is an overemphasis on the experience of same-sex attracted young men, as there is much more published literature available concerning them and their experiences. It should be taken for granted that what applies to young men may not necessarily apply to young women. Some of these differences will be highlighted where possible.

Numerous writers note that same-sex attracted young people must come to understand themselves in a society that assumes heterosexuality, provides them with scant positive information about who they are, and often reacts negatively to their enquiries. They find where they belong and how they fit within a social structure that either offers few guidelines for doing so, or tells them that they have no place (Finnegan and McNally 1987, Gibson 1994, Herdt 1989).

The development of a same-sex attracted identity usually occurs within a context of stigma. This can produce hiding, isolation, lying, maladaptive sexual patterns and even efforts to change one's orientation (Hetrick and Martin 1984). At a time when heterosexual young people are leaving home to socialize, many same-sex attracted young people are less visible, even having to hide, and are less likely to feel affirmed and supported 'or to have access to positive discourses in their peer culture about sexual difference' (Hillier *et al.* 1998: 7). Thus, some difficulties experienced are the *consequences* of being attracted to members of the same sex rather than *being* same-sex attracted, and coming out does not necessarily enhance individual well-being (Ogilvie and Brough 2000).

However, not all difficulties experienced by same-sex attracted young people who use substances are related to sexuality. There are direct and indirect associations, but it is important also to remember that young people are young people, and therefore subject to all that is involved in this transitional period of growth and development. Substance use can make sense in contexts of normal youthful experimentation (see chapter 6) with a vast array of substances to choose from, as well as the experience of accepting one's sexuality or dealing with the reactions of others to it.

Substance use among same-sex attracted young people

Western research suggests that approximately 30 per cent of same-sex attracted young people are problematic substance users (Diamond-Friedman 1990, Hall 1993, Kus 1991, Remafedi 1994), and that the rates are higher than for same-sex attracted adults. Other studies, cited in Gibson (1994), suggest that 75 per cent of same-sex attracted young people meet the criteria for a substance use disorder. Yet further research cited in this same source suggests that fewer than 20 per cent of same-sex attracted young people receiving counselling have substance use problems, but the figures are much higher for homeless gay and lesbian youth (Shifrin and Solis 1992). However, these findings tend to be overestimates due to sampling populations identified for a variety of specific issues or in specific settings – for example, homeless young people, or patrons of gay dance clubs – and may not apply to developing countries.

In order to provide a variety of data on same-sex attracted young people and their patterns of substance use, some recent Australian studies will be briefly reviewed. This does not imply that most of the research in this area is Australian, but that the available range of data provides some useful perspectives from one Western country.

In a study of over 200 gay men and over 100 lesbians aged under 24 years in the inner city area of Sydney, Bennett (1995: 19) found that alcohol consumption among his sample could 'only be described as regular and heavy'. Over 75 per cent were regular drinkers, and more than 25 per cent drank every day of the week. On an average drinking day, over 58 per cent of the young gay men and 56 per cent of the young lesbians drank more than six standard drinks, and over 18 per cent of each group drank more than twelve. When categorized, over one-third were in intermediate to high level risk categories, and over 20 per cent in the highest risk category. This was much higher than data for the general youth population.

The level of tobacco use was also high, with over 40 per cent of both males and females being categorized as heavy smokers (more than 20 cigarettes per day), and just on 60 per cent of the total sample being users of cannabis. Amyl nitrite, benzodiazepines, psychostimulants and hallucinogens were also regularly used by a substantial proportion of the sample, particularly those involved in selling or trading sex.

Other Australian studies have also tended to demonstrate high levels of substance use among same-sex attracted young people. A telephone survey of men who have sex with men (Crawford *et al.* 1998) found that of those under 20 years of age, 57.4 per cent reported use of cannabis within the last six months, compared to 41.2 per cent for the total sample. They were also more likely to have used amphetamines (22.2 per cent v. 16.5 per cent), LSD (20.4 per cent v. 10.2 per cent) and MDMA (ecstasy) (18.5 per cent v. 14.9 per cent), but less likely to have used amyl nitrite (22.2 per cent v. 30.9 per cent) and tranquillizers (4.6 per cent v. 7.8 per cent). Almost 40 per cent of the men who had injected a drug had initiated injecting drug use under the age of 20.

For the total sample, those who spent more time within the gay community and its activities were significantly more likely to use more substances (i.e. cannabis, amyl nitrite, amphetamines and ecstasy) except for heroin, than those identifying as non-gay community-attached. The HIV positive group were also significantly more likely to use larger amounts of the same group of substances than the HIV negative and untested. Men under the age of 25 were at least twice as likely to have injected than older men (Knox *et al.* 1999), and the men who injected in the last six months were significantly younger, more likely to have ever received money in exchange for sex in that six month period, and more likely to be HIV positive (about 33 per cent of the young injectors) (Crawford *et al.* 1998).

Hillier *et al.* (1998) sampled 750 same-sex attracted young people aged 14 to 21 years (mean age 18 years; 49 per cent male and 51 per cent female), mostly from the state of Victoria, Australia via advertisements in appropriate magazines, radio and the internet. Overall, they were more likely to use illegal substances than the same aged general population. More than half reported that they drank alcohol at least once a week (5 per cent daily); 30 per cent had used amphetamine-type stimulants and hallucinogens (5 per cent weekly); 62 per cent had used cannabis (7 per cent reported daily cannabis use); and 6 per cent reported the use of heroin. More females than males used these substances. Eleven per cent reported injecting drug use (15 per cent of the females and 7 per cent of the males), higher than the mean of 2–3 per cent for the state. The younger injectors (14–18 years) reported more injecting equipment sharing than the older group (19–21 years). Rural young people were more likely to be injecting drug users than those from metropolitan areas. Those who reported having been physically or verbally abused and with more confusion over their sexuality were more likely to be using heroin, cannabis and amphetamine-type stimulants. Those who were not abused and had greater support were more likely to be recreational drug users and their drug use linked to club culture.

In the Murnane *et al.* (2000) study, substance use difficulties were associated with low self-esteem, depression, anxiety, paranoia, confusion around sexuality and the stress of coming out; particular subcultures and contexts – e.g. MDMA, amphetamine-type stimulants and hallucinogen use in 'dance parties'; drug use being 'normalized' within communities of same-sex attracted young people; and drugs being integral to creating and celebrating a sense of community and belonging. There were also rural/urban, younger/older, scene/non-scene differences.

Within an Australian school population of 3,550, 6.5 per cent of respondents identified as same-sex attracted (Smith, Lindsay and Rosenthal 1999). Being same-sex attracted was associated with more frequent hazardous drinking for both young men and women than for their opposite-sex attracted peers, as well as a three- to four-fold increased likelihood of ever having injected a drug and having injected a drug in the previous twelve months. Same-sex attracted boys in Years 10 and 12 were four times more likely to have injected than other same-sex attracted boys.

These studies clearly demonstrate variability in the substance use behaviour of young people who are same-sex attracted. There are variations evident for gender, age, identification as gay/lesbian or bisexual, rural versus urban, 'clubbers' and others, and for those more victimized in relation to their sexual orientation. Substance use among same-sex attracted young people, as within the general population, is certainly not context free.

Studies from North America have yielded similar results (e.g. Faulkner and Cranston 1998, Garofalo *et al.* 1998, Noell and Ochs 2001, Orenstein 2001, Rosario, Hunter, and Gwadz 1997, Shifrin and Solis 1992). In particular, the Massachusetts Youth Risk Behavior Survey found that same-sex attracted youth (2.5 per cent of the high school sample) were more likely than peers to have engaged in multiple substance use and to have begun this behaviour earlier (Garofalo *et al.* 1998).

Recent rapid assessment and response (RAR) studies in South Eastern Europe have reflected the findings from Australia and the USA. Cucic (2002) and Wong (2002) reported RAR results from Albania, Bosnia and Herzegovina, Croatia, Federal Republic of Yugoslavia, and the Former Yugoslav Republic of Macedonia. The samples from Bosnia and Herzegovina, Macedonia and Serbia contained data on 593 young men who have sex with men. For the whole men who have sex with men sample, 35 per cent reported drug use. Of this 35 per cent, alcohol use was reported by 88 per cent, cannabis by 63 per cent, ecstasy by 27 per cent, heroin by 7 per cent, amphetamine-type stimulants by 1 per cent; 14 per cent reported that they had injected, 44 per cent shared injecting equipment, and 69 per cent (95 per cent for Bosnia and Herzegovina) had sex under the influence of drugs. About 75 per cent thought they were at risk of HIV or other sexually transmitted infections (STIs). Of those same-sex attracted men who had had sex, only 54 per cent reported regular condom use. These results were higher than for non-same-sex attracted young men sampled, but lower than for the sub-groups of young injectors and sex workers.

A recent study in Cambodia (KHANA 2003) found about 25 per cent of respondents engaging in male to male sex used alcohol or mood altering substances prior to sexual activity, especially the *pros saat*.

Some cautions

There is evidence from the published, predominantly Western, literature that young people who are same-sex attracted report levels of substance use higher than comparison general population groups. However, studies of problematic use rather than patterns of use suggest that young people who are same-sex attracted exhibit high rates because of specific cultural vulnerability such as societal oppression, internalized homophobia, stress and trauma related to coming out, under- or unemployment, and the risks associated with socializing in bars and clubs.

Many of those sampled in the studies reported to date are likely to have come from agencies working with same-sex attracted youth and urban areas with identifiable gay communities, gathering places, events or support groups. Thus, it is difficult to be sure that they actually represent the full diversity of same-sex attracted persons. The combination of drugs and sexual activity within a social context is not a recent phenomenon, or confined to the gay community and the dance party scene (Lewis and Ross 1995a and 1995b, Murnane *et al.* 2000). Savin-Williams (2001) has suggested that previous research on sexual minority youth has implicitly assumed a categorical conceptualization of sexual desire; that one is heterosexual, bisexual or homosexual. But, there are different developmental trajectories – or variability among individuals and subgroups based on biological, personal and social characteristics, and across a range of developmental milestones and transitions.

Some young people who identify as same-sex attracted during the exploratory, transitional period of adolescence may adopt a heterosexual identity and orientation in adulthood (Anhalt and Morris 1998). At times, it has been regarded as 'cool' or even fashionable by some young people to publicly identify as gay/lesbian/bisexual and androgynous. Likewise, some young people who identify as same-sex attracted may publicly 'hide' and do whatever they can to ensure that others see them as heterosexual.

Young people who know they are not heterosexual may not be prepared, either developmentally or politically, to attach themselves to culturally defined sexual categories that can have profound psychological and social ramifications. To be same-sex attracted may mean belonging to a *class* of individuals who are subject to hate crimes, prejudice and stereotypes (Hillier *et al.* 1998). In addition, most research to date has focused on young men. Young women appear to be more likely to report attraction to both sexes and bisexuality, and have been under-researched (Anhalt and Morris 1998, Hillier *et al.* 1998). There appear to be cultural and ethnic differences in same-sex attraction as well.

Risky business

Substance use is not without its negative outcomes. The harms associated with substance use identified by participants in the Murnane *et al.* (2000) study included driving under the influence of alcohol and/or other drugs; unsafe and unwanted sex; and inability to negotiate desired sex. But there are more risks than these; for example, violence and exacerbation or induction of mental disorders. Particular substances can be associated with different risks. While alcohol plays an almost ubiquitous role in risky behaviour of all types, benzodiazepines can be used to sedate and make more malleable a potential partner, and methamphetamine use has been associated with depression, psychosis and HIV-related risk behaviour (Degenhardt, Gascoigne and Howard 2002, Reback 1997).

Behaviours that may lead to HIV infection are often initiated during youth. Goodenow, Netherland and Szalacha (2002) reported on three waves of a population-based study of 3,065 male high school students in the USA, wherein 94 had male only sexual partners, and 108 had both male and female partners. Bisexuality predicted more sexual partners, unprotected intercourse, STIs and injecting drug use, as did a history of forced sex and membership of an ethnic minority. Young men with male only partners were no more risky than those with only female partners.

High risk sexual and drug-using behaviours often co-occur. Being 'high' on alcohol and/or other drugs during last sexual encounter was reported by 18.6 per cent of a sample of young urban men who have sex with men aged 15–25 years in the USA (Stueve *et al.* 2002), and 25 per cent reported unprotected anal intercourse. Gay or bisexual behaviour was an independent statistically significant predictor of drug overdose among a sample of 124 14- to 29-year-old injectors in a recent study in San Francisco (Ochoa *et al.* 2001).

Noell and Ochs (2001) found that same-sex attracted young people in the USA were more likely than other-sex attracted young people to report injecting drug use and to have recently used amphetamines, more so the young lesbian–bisexual females. It is possible that those who engage in one problem behaviour are likely to engage in other problem behaviours such as aggression, delinquency, and unsafe sexual activity (Jordan 2000). For same-sex attracted young people, and probably for those in other minority or marginalized groups, substance use is often linked with feelings of difference, with alleviation of the stress of stigmatization, to subcultures organized around bars and clubs, and where substance use can be an excuse or rationalization for risky behaviour.

Many authors have singled out methamphetamine as a substance of significant concern (McNall and Remafedi 1999). In her study of methamphetamine use among gay and bisexual men in Los Angeles, Reback (1997: ix–xv) found that participants understood 'crystal' methamphetamine 'as a functional drug that resists the social stigma associated with their sexuality, drug use and/or HIV status . . . to dissociate fears associated with sex; to cope with grief and loss; and to alleviate physical and psychological HIV-related pain'. Use of methamphetamine was often context-specific. Reback describes the experience of 'Michael', a 21-year-old Latino bisexual man, whose use of crystal in gay social settings was always associated with sexual activity, mostly unprotected; but in a heterosexual milieu it was associated with listening to music and 'kicking back' and, at times, going to find someone to fight or steal from.

Multiple substance use was associated with HIV seropositivity or unknown HIV status in a study among urban men who have sex with men in the USA by Greenwood *et al.* (2001) and Stall *et al.* (2001). Factors associated with multiple drug use included being younger, HIV positive status, having a family history of substance use, substance use being perceived as a positive tension reduction mechanism, greater gay bar/club attendance, multiple sex partners, and not being in a steady relationship. The authors suggest that connection to gay culture can be protective or risk enhancing, and found that heavy and/or problematic substance use is complex and grounded in multiple levels: the individual, including demographic factors, early adverse life circumstances and current mental health concerns, the interpersonal and the socio-cultural. It also 'requires an understanding of MSM [men who have sex with men] sexual cultures, perhaps as an expression of a conjoined "high-risk" or "sensation-seeking" life-style' (Stall *et al.* 2001: 1599).

The possible role of delinquency and substance use as mediators of risky sexual behaviour has been identified (Winters, Remafedi and Chan 1996), as alcohol and other drugs have disinhibiting effects, and/or decrease pain and/or increase arousal. Young male sex workers in Oslo, Norway have been reported as using more drugs (especially alcohol and heroin), and were also more likely to have conduct/delinquency problems and been victims of violence, than their non-sex worker peers (Pederson and Hegna 2003). However, delinquent behaviour usually pre-dates substance use in those where it co-exists.

In relation to minority status, Lemp *et al.* (1994), in their sample of young men recruited in public venues, found that HIV positive status was high (9.4 per cent), but higher (21.2 per cent) for young African-Americans. Most of the young HIV positive men did not know their HIV serostatus. The influence of nitrites and/or alcohol during sex was associated with unprotected anal intercourse, but this may be either causal or a marker of 'lifestyle among persons at high risk'. Doherty *et al.* (2000) found sexual practices associated with HIV included reporting more than 100 lifetime sex partners, a history of sexual assault, being gay or bisexual, trading sex for money or drugs after starting to inject, and starting injecting younger. However, some of these could be markers for other risky practices as well and thus there is a need for a broad profile of risk and sexual orientation.

Luna (1997) has documented some of the stories of young people, mostly from California, USA who are HIV positive, and highlights the role of amphetamine-type stimulants in risky behaviour. He quotes José, a 22-year-old, gay-identified Latino who is HIV positive:

> Cocaine, crack, everything except heroin. Crystal meth, I shot up three times. Crystal meth, pot – it's boring though. It just makes you sleepy and tired; all you want to do is eat and go to sleep. With crystal, you don't eat for days. Talk about a great way to diet. Forget Jenny Craig, just shoot up crystal. . . . Have a couple of lines before a meal, forget the Slimfast shake. . . . A vacuum cleaner couldn't clean better than a person on speed. . . . Gosh, but then the five days afterward are depression and loneliness, oh! . . . what goes up that high, comes down that low.
>
> (p. 7)

Others have identified the complex connections between substance use and elevated risk of suicidal behaviour among same-sex attracted young people. In a study of over 400 US young people aged 18 to 30 years, of mean age 21 years, recruited in a study of suicidal behaviour and its correlates among same-sex attracted and heterosexual young people, approximately 45 per cent of the sample identified as same-sex attracted (Howard *et al.* 2002, Nicholas and Howard 1998). Having made a suicide attempt was reported by 20.9 per cent of the gay males and 29.3 per cent of the lesbians.

Analysis revealed that male same-sex attracted suicide attempters were significantly more likely than gay male non-attempters to have received less support from their families, had experienced more verbal violence and more unwanted sexual contact after the age of 16, and had used more amphetamines and inhalants recently. Female same-sex attracted suicide attempters were significantly more likely than lesbian non-attempters to have received less support from their families, and experienced more verbal and physical violence and more unwanted sexual contact before the age of 16. Around the time of the decision to make a suicide attempt, alcohol and cannabis were the most widely used substances, and alcohol was the substance used to make the attempt easier.

Fergusson, Horwood and Beautrais (1999) from their New Zealand longitudinal study also found that those identifying as gay, lesbian or bisexual had increased risk of depression, generalized anxiety disorder, conduct disorder, substance use/dependence, suicidal ideation and attempts.

Overall, there appear to be significant negative outcomes associated with substance use for same-sex attracted young people; particularly in unwanted and unsafe sex, HIV infection and suicidality. Attachment to gay subculture has been identified as both protective and risky. However, the cautions raised previously also apply, as many studies arise from samples that were recruited from settings where higher risk behaviour or enhanced vulnerability may be evident, and not all same-sex attracted young people are equally vulnerable or 'at risk'.

Why the elevated risk?

For some same-sex attracted youth, external and internalized homophobia, perceived negative reactions from friends and/or family after coming out, or homelessness may result in the onset of depression, suicidal thoughts and behaviour, and substance use (Plummer 1999, Safren and Heimberg 1999, Savin-Williams 1994). Same-sex attracted young people often experience elevated levels of verbal and physical violence from both family and peers (Garofalo *et al.* 1998 and 1999, Hershberger and D'Augelli 1995, Remafedi 1990, Hunter 1990). This can be particularly so for young people who openly identify as same-sex attracted, and/or who present with gender atypical appearance and behaviour (Brown, Chadwick and Goldflam 1999). The Massachusetts Youth Risk Behavior Survey found that same-sex attracted young people were more likely than peers to have been victimized or threatened, to have suicidal ideation and made attempts, and to report multiple substance use and sexual risk behaviour (Garofalo *et al.* 1998).

For gay and lesbian young people, the increased risk of substance use is mediated by stress caused by the contradiction of needing to establish an integrated sense of self, while doing so runs the risk of peer and family rejection, fears for personal safety, and the ongoing experience of homophobic remarks and 'jokes' that are common in high schools. Coming out is unique to young people who are same-sex attracted (Anhalt and Morris 1998). By contrast, heterosexual youth develop their sexual identity in the context of a societal norm where sexual milestones such as 'the first kiss' are discussed openly with peers and often looked on with pride. The first sexual experience of same-sex attracted youth can be furtive, anonymous and/or with an older partner and 'medicated' by one or more substances. Such experiences may leave some unsure of the normality and acceptability of their experience.

It could be argued that most gays/lesbians with substance use problems appear to be ambivalent about or attempt to hide their sexuality. Gibson (1994) has suggested that:

> Substance use often begins in early adolescence when youth first experience conflicts around their sexual orientation. It initially serves the functional purposes of reducing the pain and anxiety of external

conflicts and reducing the internal inhibitions of homosexual feelings and behaviour.

(p. 21)

Thus, substance use can medicate anxiety related to concealing one's identity, help to discharge sexual impulses more comfortably, act as an antidote to the pain of exclusion, ridicule and rejection, and can provide a feeling of power and self-worth to counteract feeling devalued. However, substance dependence can in time become another form of oppression.

Minority status may also play a role in increased vulnerability to the development of substance use-related difficulties (Anhalt and Morris 1998). One hundred and thirty-one primarily Hispanic and Black US 14- to 19-year-old gay and bisexual males were surveyed by Rotheram-Borus *et al.* (1994). Rates of substance use were higher among this sample than among young men in a 1991 national household survey. For example, lifetime prevalence rates were one and a half times higher for alcohol, two times higher for cannabis, and thirteen times higher for cocaine. Use of alcohol, cannabis or cocaine at least once a week was approximately three to fifteen times higher among young people in this sample. However, gay/bisexual identification may be a more critical factor than ethnicity in placing youth at risk for HIV (Solorio, Swendeman and Rotheram-Borus 2003).

In addition, differences between Puerto Rican, Cuban and Mexican young men have been reported. Younger men are more likely to identify as bisexual than those in their twenties. Differing explanations are offered. For example, in a study of US Latino men, Diaz (1998) found HIV risk was higher for drug users. He posits that

risky behaviour may occur in situations where the sexual activity of Latino gay and bisexual men is disconnected from personal conscious control (through the influence of alcohol and drugs) and disconnected from interpersonal relations and interaction and negotiation (through anonymous sex in public environments).

(p. 46)

The work of Schifter (2000) also highlights the differences between a variety of private and public enactments of sexuality, and the role of drugs to make money and enact alternative and desired sexualities among apparently heterosexual men who have sex with men.

For others, sexual orientation may play a more distal role; its relationship to risk behaviour may be complex and associated with factors such as difficulties with a partner and/or a sense of isolation from previous support structures such as from peers and family (Hart and Heimberg 2001). Thus, it may erode the possible benefits of what might be protective factors for most young people. Their isolation may be reinforced by a fear of discussing

their possible confusion and concerns. Substance use, while possibly associated with celebrations, socializing and/or attempts to self-medicate negative
feelings or memories, tends to increase the risk of deliberate self-harm
significantly.

Common explanations for these high levels of substance use include the
role of various substances in medicating the effects of coming out, alienation
and harassment (Rosario, Hunter and Gwadz 1997), celebrating coming out
(Murnane *et al.* 2000), and the role of gay bars as the only readily available
arena in which same-sex attracted young people can socialize (Bennett 1995):
'Historically in both Australia and other developed countries, drug use has
been at the centre of the establishment and the "coming out" of the gay and
lesbian community as a whole' (Murnane *et al.* 2000: 11).

Gay bars are seen as a major contributor to increased use of substances by
young and older same-sex attracted people, as they provide a place to feel
safe, to socialize and find partners. Diamond-Friedman (1990) reported that
49 per cent of gay men and 28 per cent of lesbians interviewed frequented
bars once to twice a week in the twelve months prior to interview in the USA.
In an Australian study, Bennett (1995) found that over 80 per cent of his
sample frequented gay/lesbian/mixed bars at least once per week, with about
17 per cent being daily attenders. There was a correlation between making
a decision about sexual identity and beginning to go to bars. Over 60 per
cent of the gay men and 50 per cent of the lesbians went to a gay/lesbian/
mixed bar before their 18th birthdays. Gay bars can be seen as providing a
family and an alternative form of social support, places to celebrate, places
to test one's new identity, and even places to be political (Bennett 1995). Kus
(1988 and 1991), however, provides an alternative account, feeling that some
young people 'explode out' rather than come out. They may do this in riskier
contexts such as bars, clubs or public sex venues.

What assistance can be provided?

Safety, support and information are crucial. But it should not be assumed
that all same-sex attracted young people who are using substances require
programmes or, if they do, same-sex attracted specific ones. Nor are all
interventions the domain of the medical profession or other allied health
professions. Everyone in civil society has a role to play, including families,
schools and communities.

For those who require treatment, it needs to be acknowledged that substance use treatment settings can be oppressive and discriminatory and often
favour heterosexist views of the world and behaviour, with homosexuality
being seen as pathological and/or something to be feared. In these kinds
of contexts, same-sex attracted young people can become scapegoats and
a distraction or diversion (MacEwan 1994, Ratner 1988). When same-
sex attracted young people sense rejection, alienation or discomfort they

may deal with them by acting-out or -up. This becomes self-defeating ultimately, but at least discharges some distress and confirms the view that others
will only reject them and/or that they are not worthy or too different to be
understood.

Exposure to a range of role models may decrease isolation by providing
examples of resilience and coping. However, the available range of roles for
same-sex attracted young people is limited and can be stereotypical. For
example, gay men are often portrayed as effeminate, drag queens, or as
having AIDS (Sullivan and Schneider 1987), and unlike other young people
in minority groups, the fathers of gay adolescents do not prepare their sons
to be gay, nor can they communicate what it is like to be gay (Dank 1971).
At most, their fathers can accept and support their identity. Should this
support not be offered or received, it is possible that the same-sex attracted
young person may feel more isolated and vulnerable. This may be more so
in developing countries and those in contexts where stigma and the social
'invisibility' of same-sex attracted people are common.

Parents clearly need support in such situations, but may not know where
or how to access information or assistance, or may be too embarrassed to
do so. Resources which may assist parents and friends are available,
including literature (Western Australia AIDS Council 1997a), websites and
organizations such as *Someone You Love*, an information booklet developed
in Western Australia by PFLAG (Parents and Friends of Lesbians and Gays).

Anecdotal evidence suggests that same-sex attracted youth will often
read about homosexuality prior to coming out. Data collected by the Reach
Out! on-line suicide prevention service found that a gay-identified website
was a major referrer (Morrison and Sullivan 2002). This indicates that same-
sex attracted young people, like others, frequently access the internet, an
anonymous source of information and connection with other young people
exploring their sexuality. Making relevant web addresses readily available in
a variety of settings, such as general practitioners' surgeries and youth centres,
via posters and brochures, can be helpful. While there has been an increase
in groups and resources for same-sex attracted people in developing and
transitional countries (e.g. in India, China, Thailand, the Philippines, Russia
and Latin America), many young people questioning their sexuality access
Western sites. However, this can be problematic as many such sites primarily
cater to Western young people, with few language or literacy difficulties.

Schools and other agencies can also play a major role in providing information and support. Some argue that schools should develop special support
roles and structures, such as diversity rooms and diversity room specialists
(Nichols 1999), and psycho-educational services (Safren and Heimberg
1999). In relation to work with same-sex attracted young people, workers
need to honestly check for homophobia both within themselves and within
their agencies. Reading in the area, bringing issues up in staff and other
meetings, challenging biases and prejudice, and feeling more confident in

raising relevant issues with clients will better inform future work with such young people.

In relation to any treatment interventions, there are some areas that require attention. These include dealing with the possible stress connected with management of a same-sex attracted identity; disrupted peer relationships; the decision to disclose to family and the consequences of this; the emotional reactions to developing close relationships; possible isolation from same-sex attracted affirming situations; discrimination, harassment and violence due to sexual orientation; and anxieties about sexual behaviour, especially HIV, other blood-borne viruses and STIs.

Conclusions

Substance use and sexuality are related to one another in complex ways. As for most young people, there are variations in patterns and extent of use, and exposure to risk varies according to age, gender, location, psychopathology unrelated to sexuality and attachment to various subcultures. Sexuality issues may also play a distal or proximal role in the development of substance use and associated difficulties. There is evidence that some same-sex attracted youth are at elevated risk for HIV and other blood-borne viruses and STIs, and suicide attempts, but not as yet for claims that they are over-represented in completed suicide figures. As yet, there is little information about girls and young women. This area needs urgent attention.

While discussion and debate about these matters has begun, more attention needs to be given to the consequences of globalization and appropriation or insertion of Western terms such as gay, lesbian and queer into developing and other cultures. Likewise, preventive or other interventions need to be mindful of broad national, local, cultural and religious contexts, and should not exacerbate any potential negative outcomes.

Most same-sex attracted young people appear to come through the period of adolescence minimally scarred and resilient; a minority do not. The development of environments, both interpersonal and structural, that support and offer protection to young people has the potential to make a significant impact in the lives of same-sex attracted young people. Otherwise, some may feel that being drugged or dead are preferable options to being same-sex attracted.

References

Aggleton, P. (ed.) (1999) *Men Who Sell Sex: International Perspectives on Male Prostitution and HIV/AIDS*, London: UCL Press.

Anhalt, K. and Morris, T. (1998) 'Developmental and adjustment issues of gay, lesbian, and bisexual adolescents: a review of the empirical literature', *Clinical Child and Family Psychology Review*, 1: 215–30.

Bennett, G. (1995) *Young and Gay: A Study of Gay Youth in Sydney*, Sydney: Twenty-Ten Association.

Bondyopadhyay, A. and Khan, S. (2004) *Against the Odds: The Impact of Legal, Socio-cultural, Legislative and Socio-economic Impediments to Effective HIV/AIDS Intervention with Males Who Have Sex with Males in Bangladesh*, Bangladesh: Bandu and NAZ Foundation International.

Brown, G., Chadwick, R. and Goldflam, A. (1999) *Here for Life Youth Sexuality Project – Evaluation and Final Report*, Perth: Western Australia AIDS Council.

Crawford, J., Kippax, S., Rodden, P., Donohoe, S. and Van de Ven, P. (1998) *Male Call '96: National Telephone Survey of Men Who Have Sex With Men*, Sydney: National Centre in HIV Social Research, Macquarie University.

Cucic, V. (2002) *Rapid Assessment and Response on HIV/AIDS among Especially Vulnerable Young People in Serbia*, Belgrade: UNICEF.

Dank, B. (1971) 'Coming out in the gay world', *Psychiatry*, 34: 180–97.

Davies, P., Hickson, F., Weatherburn, P. and Hunt, A. (1993) *Sex, Gay Men and AIDS*, London: Falmer Press.

Degenhardt, L., Gascoigne, M. and Howard, J. (2002) 'Young people's drug use when heroin is less available', *Youth Studies Australia*, 21: 11–16.

Diamond-Friedman, C. (1990) 'A multivariant model of alcoholism specific to gay–lesbian populations', *Alcoholism Quarterly*, 7: 111–17.

Diaz, R. (1998) *Latino Gay Men and HIV: Culture, Sexuality and Risk Behaviour*, New York: Routledge.

Doherty, M., Garfein, R., Monterroso, E., Brown, D. and Vlahov, D. (2000) 'Correlates of HIV infection among young adult short-term injection drug users', *AIDS*, 14: 717–26.

Faulkner, A. and Cranston, K. (1998) 'Correlates of same-sex sexual behavior in a random sample of Massachusetts high school students', *American Journal of Public Health*, 88: 262–6.

Fergusson, D.M., Horwood, L.J. and Beautrais, A.L. (1999) 'Is sexual orientation related to mental health problems and suicidality in young people?', *Archives of General Psychiatry*, 56: 876–80.

Finnegan, D. and McNally, E. (1987) *Dual Identities: Counselling Chemically Dependent Gay Men and Lesbians*, Center City, MN: Hazeldon.

Garofalo, R., Wolf, R., Kessel, S., Palfrey, J. and DuRant, R. (1998) 'The association between health risk behaviors and sexual orientation among a school-based sample of adolescents', *Pediatrics*, 101: 895–902.

Garofalo, R., Wolf, R., Lawrence, M., Wissow, S., Woods, E. and Goodman, E. (1999) 'Sexual orientation and risk of suicide attempts among a representative sample of youth', *Archives of Pediatric and Adolescent Medicine*, 153: 487–93.

Gibson, P. (1994) 'Gay male and lesbian youth suicide', in G. Remafedi (ed.) *Death by Denial: Studies of Suicide in Gay and Lesbian Teenagers*, Boston: Aylson.

Goodenow, C., Netherland, J. and Szalacha, L. (2002) 'AIDS-related risk among adolescent males who have sex with males, females, or both: evidence from a statewide survey', *American Journal of Public Health*, 92: 203–10.

Gosine, A. and Binswanger, H. (2004) 'Sexual minorities, violence and HIV/AIDS: the response in the developing world', paper prepared for UNAIDS, UNESCAP, World Bank Pre-conference Symposium on Sexual Minorities and HIV, Bangkok, July.

Greenwood, G., Whire, E., Page-Shafer, K., Bien, E., Osmond, D., Paul, J. and Stall, R. (2001) 'Correlates of heavy substance use among young gay and bisexual men: the San Francisco Young Men's Health Study', *Drug and Alcohol Dependence*, 61: 105–12.

Hall, J. (1993) 'Lesbians and alcohol: patterns and paradoxes in medical notions and lesbians' beliefs', *Journal of Psychoactive Drugs*, 25: 109–19.

Hart, T. and Heimberg, R. (2001) 'Presenting problems among treatment seeking gay, lesbian and bisexual youth', *Journal of Clinical Psychology*, 57: 615–27.

Herdt, G. (1989) 'Introduction: gay and lesbian youth, emergent identities, and cultural scenes at home and abroad', *Journal of Homosexuality*, 17: 1–42.

Hershberger, S.L. and D'Augelli, A.R. (1995) 'The impact of victimization on the mental health and suicidality of lesbian, gay and bisexual youth', *Developmental Psychology*, 31: 65–74.

Hetrick, E. and Martin, D. (1984) 'Ego dystonic homosexuality: a developmental view', in E. Hetrick and T. Stein (eds) *Innovations in Psychotherapy with Homosexuals*, Washington: American Psychiatric Press.

Hillier, L., Dempsey, D., Harrison, L., Beale, L., Matthews, L. and Rosenthal, D. (1998) *Writing Themselves in: A National Report on the Sexuality, Health and Well-Being of Same-Sex Attracted Young People*, Melbourne: Centre for the Study of Sexually Transmissible Diseases, National Centre in HIV Social Research, La Trobe University.

Howard, J., Nicholas, J., Brown, G. and Karacanta, A. (2002) 'Same-sex attracted youth and suicide', in L. Rowling, G. Martin and L. Walker (eds) *Mental Health Promotion and Young People*, Sydney: McGraw-Hill.

Hunter, J. (1990) 'Violence against lesbian and gay male youth', *Journal of Interpersonal Violence*, 5: 295–300.

Jordan, K. (2000) 'Substance abuse among gay, lesbian, bisexual, transgender, and questioning adolescents', *School Psychology Review*, 29: 201–6.

Khan, S. (1999) 'Through a window darkly: men who sell sex to men in India and Bangladesh', in P. Aggleton (ed.) *Men Who Sell Sex*, London: UCL Press.

KHANA and the International HIV/AIDS Alliance (2003) *Out of the Shadows: Male to Male Sexual Behaviour in Cambodia*, Phnom Penh: KHANA.

Knox, S., Kippax, S., Crawford, J., Prestage, G. and Van De Ven, P. (1999) 'Non-prescription drug use by gay men in Sydney, Melbourne and Brisbane', *Drug and Alcohol Review*, 18: 425–33.

Kus, R. (1988) 'Alcoholism and non-acceptance of gay self: the critical link', in M. Ross (ed.) *The Treatment of Homosexuals with Mental Health Disorders*, New York: Harrington.

Kus, R. (1991) 'Sobriety, friends, and gay men', *Archives of Psychiatry*, V(3), 171–7.

Lemp, G., Hirozawa, A., Givertz, D., Nieri, G., Anderson, L., Lindegren, M., Janssen, R. and Katz, M. (1994) 'Seroprevalence of HIV and risk behaviors among young homosexual and bisexual men: the San Francisco/Berkeley Young Men's Survey', *Journal of the American Medical Association*, 272: 449–54.

Lewis, L. and Ross, M. (1995a) 'The gay dance party culture in Sydney: a qualitative analysis', *Journal of Homosexuality*, 29: 41–70.

Lewis, L. and Ross, M. (1995b) *A Select Body: The Gay Dance Party Subculture and the HIV/AIDS Pandemic*, London: Cassell.

Luna, G. Cajetan (1997) *Youths Living with HIV: Self-evident Truths*, New York: Harrington.

MacEwan, I. (1994) 'Differences in assessment and treatment approaches for homosexual clients', *Drug and Alcohol Review*, 13(1): 57–62.

McNall, M. and Remafedi, G. (1999) 'Relationship of amphetamine and other substance use to unprotected intercourse among young men who have sex with men', *Archives of Pediatric Adolescent Medicine*, 153: 1130–5.

Morrison, M. and Sullivan, C. (2002) 'Using the net to engage youth in mental health promotion: the Reach Out! experience', in L. Rowling, G. Martin and L. Walker (eds) *Mental Health Promotion and Young People*, Sydney: McGraw Hill.

Murnane, A., Smith, A., Crompton, L., Snow, P. and Munro, G. (2000) *Beyond Perceptions: A Report on Alcohol and Other Drug Use among Gay, Lesbian, Bisexual and Queer Communities in Victoria*, Melbourne: ALSO Foundation, Centre for Youth Drug Studies and Vic. Health.

Nicholas, J. and Howard, J. (1998) 'Better dead than gay? Depression, suicide ideation and attempt among a sample of gay- and straight-identified males aged 18–24', *Youth Studies Australia*, 17: 28–33.

Nichols, S. (1999) 'Gay, lesbian, and bisexual youth: understanding diversity and promoting tolerance in schools', *The Elementary School Journal*, 99: 505–14.

Noell, J. and Ochs, L. (2001) 'Relationship of sexual orientation to substance use, suicidal ideation, suicide attempts, and other factors in a population of homeless adolescents', *Journal of Adolescent Health*, 29: 31–6.

Ochoa, K., Hahn, J., Seal, K. and Moss, A. (2001) 'Overdosing among young injection drug users in San Francisco', *Addictive Behaviors*, 26: 453–60.

Ogilvie, V. and Brough, M. (2000) *Our Pathway 'Out': Growing up Gay – Dealing with Life Stress – and Coping*, Brisbane: Youth and Family Services (Logan City) Inc., Queensland Health.

Orenstein, A. (2001) 'Substance use among gay and lesbian adolescents', *Journal of Homosexuality*, 41: 1–15.

Pederson, W. and Hegna, K. (2003) 'Children and adolescents who sell sex: a community study', *Social Science and Medicine*, 56: 135–47.

Plummer, D. (1999) *One of the Boys: Masculinity, Homophobia and Modern Manhood*, New York: Harrington Park Press.

Ratner, E. (1988) 'A model for the treatment of lesbian and gay alcohol abusers', *Alcohol Quarterly*, 5: 25–44.

Reback, C. (1997) *The Social Construction of a Gay Drug: Methamphetamine use among Gay and Bisexual Males*, Los Angeles: City of Los Angeles, AIDS Prevention Division.

Remafedi, G. (1990) 'Fundamental issues in the care of homosexual youth', *Medical Clinics of North America*, 74: 1169–79.

Remafedi, G. (1994) 'Predictors of unprotected intercourse among gay and bisexual youth: knowledge, beliefs and behavior', *Pediatrics*, 94: 163–8.

Rosario, M., Hunter, J. and Gwadz, M. (1997) 'Exploration of substance use among lesbian, gay and bisexual youth: prevalence and correlates', *Journal of Adolescent Research*, 12: 454–76.

Rotherum-Borus, M.J., Hunter, J. and Rosario, M. (1994) 'Suicidal behavior and gay related stress among gay and bisexual adolescents', *Journal of Adolescent Research*, 9: 498–508.

Safren, S. and Heimberg, R. (1999) 'Depression, hopelessness, suicidality, and related factors in sexual minority and heterosexual adolescents', *Journal of Consulting and Clinical Psychology*, 67: 859–66.

Savin-Williams, R. (1994) 'Verbal and physical abuse as stressors in the lives of lesbian, gay male and bisexual youths: associations with school problems, running away, substance abuse, prostitution and suicide', *Journal of Consulting and Clinical Psychology*, 62: 261–9.

Savin-Williams, R. (2001) 'A critique of research on sexual-minority youth', *Journal of Adolescence*, 24: 5–13.

Schifter, J. (2000) *Public Sex in a Latin Society*, New York: Haworth Hispanic.

Seattle Department of School Education (1995) *Youth Risk Behavior Survey, Seattle, WA data summary*, http://www.virtualcity.com/youthsuicide/gbsuicide.htm.

Shifrin, F. and Solis, M. (1992) 'Chemical dependency in gay and lesbian youth', *Journal of Chemical Dependency Treatment*, 5: 67–76.

Smith, A., Lindsay, J. and Rosenthal, D. (1999) 'Same-sex attraction, drug injection and binge drinking among Australian adolescents', *Australian and New Zealand Journal of Public Health*, 23: 643–6.

Solorio, R., Swendeman, D. and Rotheram-Borus, M. (2003) 'Risk among young gay and bisexual men living with HIV', *AIDS Education and Prevention*, 15 (1 Suppl. A): 80–9.

Stall, R., Paul, J., Greenwood, G., Pollack, L., Bein, E., Crosby, M., Mills, T., Binson, D., Coates, T. and Catania, J. (2001) 'Alcohol use, drug use and alcohol-related problems among men who have sex with men: the Urban Men's Health Study', *Addiction*, 96: 1589–601.

Stueve, A., O'Donnell, L., Duran, R., San Doval, A., Geier, J. (Community Intervention Trial for Youth Study Team) (2002) 'Being high and taking sexual risks: findings from a multisite survey of urban young men who have sex with men', *AIDS Education and Prevention*, 14: 482–95.

Sullivan, T. and Schneider, M. (1987) 'Development and identity issues in adolescent homosexuality', *Child and Adolescent Social Work*, 4: 13–23.

Western Australia AIDS Council (1997a) *Someone You Love*, Perth: Western Australia AIDS Council.

Western Australia AIDS Council (1997b) *You're Not Alone*, Perth: Western Australia AIDS Council.

Winters, K., Remafedi, G. and Chan, B. (1996) 'Assessing drug abuse among gay–bisexual young men', *Psychology of Addictive Behaviours*, 10: 228–36.

Wong, E. (2002) *Rapid Assessment and Response on HIV/AIDS among Especially Vulnerable Young People in South Eastern Europe*, Belgrade: UNICEF.

Chapter 8

Drinking behaviour, coming of age and risk

Sandra Bullock and Robin Room

Drinking alcohol, and experiencing its intoxicating effects, are fairly universal phenomena among the young people of the world. In this chapter, we touch on three broad questions. What do we know about the alcohol consumption patterns of young people around the world? Second, how has the consumption of alcohol by young people been conceptualized in the literature? Finally, how does drinking relate to other risk activities of young adults, such as violence and sex? Given the quantity of information that is present in the literature and the limited space available, we do not attempt to provide an exhaustive overview of the literature in response to these three questions but merely highlight selected areas of it.

Our emphasis here is on young people's drinking, particularly in relation to sexuality, but it should be recognized that drinking by young people generally reflects the context of adult drinking norms and drinking-related behaviour in a particular culture. Within Europe, for instance, there is a fairly close relationship between the predominance of intoxication in the drinking of 15 year-olds and the predominance of intoxication in the general patterns of adult drinking in society (Room, 2003). It has been argued that it is a mistake to adopt countermeasures to youth drinking without considering also measures for the adult population (Bonnie and O'Connell, 2004: 98–9), if only because young people are likely to see as hypocritical a message to 'Do what I say, not what I do'.

In general, much more is known of alcohol patterns and the cultural position of drinking in the developed countries than is known of its use in the developing world. Anthropological studies of the aspects of alcohol in relation to culture and social life in tribal societies and villages date often from decades ago and are thus largely out of date (Room *et al.*, 2002). The relative availability of alcohol to a population, and its young people in particular, depends in part on economic factors; as societies become more developed, alcohol becomes more readily available, and its use and abuse tends to increase. What limited information is available with respect to patterns of alcohol use and resulting harms in the developing world is largely based upon the more affluent, westernized segments of the population, and is probably not representative of populations as a whole (Room *et al.*, 2002). Thus, reflecting the available data, this chapter will focus more heavily upon drinking patterns in developed countries.

Young people and alcohol consumption – global patterns

An individual's propensity for drinking, and problem drinking in particular, is at least partially rooted in biological and genetic factors; however, drinking does not occur in isolation. Drinking behaviour is highly influenced by societal norms and the behavioural patterns of those around youth, ranging from their closest interpersonal relationships (including parents and peers) to societal-level structural forces and barriers. Thus, in discussing youth alcohol consumption, we refer to differences in patterns and levels of consumption within and between countries and sub-cultures. In considering drinking cultures and patterns, the number of dimensions available for comparison is quite large. This section focuses upon abstention, frequency of heavy drinking, the relationship between heavy drinking and drinking episodes in general, and attitudes concerning the acceptance of drinking and intoxication by youth.

Derived primarily from population surveys, the data in Table 8.1 show the estimated rates of life-long abstention (never consumed a drink of an alcoholic beverage) from alcohol consumption by young people in the 14 world sub-regions as defined by the WHO (Rehm *et al.*, 2004). There are substantial proportions of youth populations in both developing societies and Islamic regions that have never consumed alcohol. Lifelong abstention rates are high for young men, and even higher for young women in the Middle East and South-East Asia. Rates are moderate for young men and high for young women in Africa, and low for young men, but high for young women, in East Asia. In other regions, the abstention rates for males are low and females low to moderate. Latin America is the only developing region where the reported rates of abstention are similar to those in the developed regions. Not seen in this table is that these regional rates of abstention for young people do not appear to differ from those of middle aged adults in the same regions, reflecting the strong interpersonal and cultural influences on consumption (Rehm *et al.*, 2004).

Cross-national surveys, such as the study of Health Behaviour in School-aged Children (HBSC), provide more detailed and comparable information within primarily developed countries. Students aged 11 to 15 years were asked whether they had ever tasted an alcoholic drink, how often they drank a range of alcoholic beverages and how often, if ever, they drank enough alcohol that they became really drunk (Gabhainn and François, 2000; Schmid and Gabhainn, 2004). Results for those aged 15 are shown in Table 8.2. By the age of 15, Israeli girls are far less likely to have tried alcohol than

Table 8.1 Estimated percentage abstinence from alcohol consumption of
population aged 15–29, by sex and World Health Organization (WHO)
sub-region

Sub-region[a]	per cent abstainers – last year		Hazardous drinking pattern[b]
	males	females	
AFR-D			
(e.g., Nigeria, Algeria)	51.0	74.6	2.5
AFR-E			
(e.g., Ethiopia, South Africa)	43.2	71.5	3.1
AMR-A			
(e.g., Canada, Cuba, USA)	24.0	36.0	2.0
AMR-B			
(e.g., Brazil, Mexico)	22.0	46.3	3.1
AMR-D			
(e.g., Bolivia, Peru)	29.8	43.1	3.1
EMR-B			
(e.g., Iran, Saudi Arabia)	78.9	93.7	2.0
EMR-D			
(e.g., Afghanistan, Pakistan)	89.8	97.5	2.4
EUR-A			
(e.g., Germany, France, UK)	7.4	13.8	1.3
EUR-B			
(e.g., Armenia, Poland, Turkey)	23.7	41.0	2.9
EUR-C			
(e.g., Russia, Ukraine)	8.8	14.0	3.6
SEAR-B			
(e.g., Indonesia, Thailand)	63.1	88.5	2.5
SEAR-D			
(e.g., Bangladesh, India)	71.7	93.7	3.0
WPR-A			
(e.g., Australia, Japan)	9.5	16.3	1.2
WPR-B			
(e.g., China, Philippines, Vietnam)	15.3	67.4	2.2

Source: Rehm *et al.*, 2004: 982–5.

Notes:
(a) A full list of countries included in each WHO sub-region can be seen in Rehm *et al.* 2004:
973–9.
(b) Pattern values are defined as follows: units range between 1 and 4; regional averages are
population-weighted country averages for the population aged 15 years and older.
Definitions of the extreme categories of risk factor levels: Level 1: based on score of initial
values reflecting least detrimental patterns of drinking such as least heavy drinking
occasions, drinking with meals, no fiesta drinking and least drinking in public places. Level
4: based on score of initial pattern components with highest values reflecting detrimental
patterns such as many heavy drinking occasions, drinking outside of meals, high level of
fiesta drinking and drinking in public places.

any other group. While more Israeli 15 year-old boys have abstained than boys from other countries, the difference is not as substantial as seen with girls. In virtually all other countries studied, the gender differences seen at age 11 (girls more likely to be abstinent) are actually quite small by the age of 15. This is opposite to the pattern seen later in life, and may reflect that adolescent females mature at a more rapid rate than males, and tend to date and socialize with males older than themselves (Wheeler and Cunter, 1987). Abstinence in the developed countries falls quite rapidly between the ages of 11 and 15 (Gabhainn and François, 2000). In fact, the average age of alcohol debut among those asked when they were 15 in these countries was age 12.3 (SD 2.3) for boys and 12.9 (SD 1.9) for girls (Schmid and Gabhainn, 2004).

While rates of abstinence do not differ very much between boys and girls by the age of 15, drinking patterns do. Boys are more likely to drink alcohol more regularly, and are even more likely to drink for the purpose of becoming drunk in most countries than girls. The centre set of columns in Table 8.2 shows the percentage of HBSC 15 year-olds who reported drinking alcohol at least weekly, by country. In all countries studied, boys were more likely than girls to report getting drunk (right-hand column of Table 8.2); however, there is some evidence that the gender gap is decreasing (Gabhainn and François, 2000; Johnston, O'Malley and Bachman, 1991; Schmid and Gabhainn, 2004). For both boys and girls, beer was the most popular drink. However, students in Wales, England and Greece were among the highest spirits consumers, and French students were more likely to drink wine frequently, emulating the adult drinking cultures in these countries (Gabhainn and François, 2000). It should be noted that the countries in which young people drink more frequently are generally not the same countries that have a high proportion of their youth experiencing drunkenness at an early age. While young people from most Nordic countries are among the most likely to experience drunkenness, they are much less likely to drink regularly. An exception to this is seen with youth from the United Kingdom and Denmark: they are likely to already have been drunk by the age of 15 and yet also drink weekly. Overall, time trends suggest that youth alcohol consumption has increased in most countries over the last 30–35 years (with a decrease during the 1980s and early 1990s), and similar trends are also seen for heavy episodic (binge) drinking among youth and young adults (Gabhainn and François, 2000; Johnston, O'Malley and Bachman, 2002a; Johnston, O'Malley and Bachman, 2002b; Schmid and Gabhainn, 2004; Windle, 1999).

While there have been many surveys of drinking among young people in developing countries (Jernigan, 2001:14–38), the data are not often collected and reported in comparable form. As with drinking among adults in developing countries, a common pattern is that abstinence is more common than in most developed societies, but on the other hand intoxication is often quite common among young people who drink at all. For instance, only 34 per

Table 8.2 Drinking patterns of 15 year-olds, from Health Behaviour in School-aged Children (HBSC) Studies 1997/1998 and 2001/2002

Geographic location/country (hazardous drinking score)[a]	Prevalence of abstention[b] 1997/98[c]			Prevalence of weekly drinking 2001/2[d]			Prevalence of being drunk 2 or more times 2001/2[d]		
	females (%)	males (%)	rank	females (%)	males (%)	rank	females (%)	males (%)	rank
Nordic Countries									
Denmark (2)	4	5	19	44	50	5	65	68	1
Finland (3)	5	6	15	16	18	30	56	53	5
Greenland (–)	6	10	9	11	29	26	53	64	3
Norway (3)	14	16	3	19	20	24	41	39	11
Sweden (3)	5	4	16	17	23	23	38	40	14
United Kingdom and Ireland									
England (2)	4	4	20	48	56	2	55	55	4
Ireland (3)	6	7	13	16	20	29	32	33	21
Scotland (2)	2	2	23	42	44	6	52	52	7
Wales (2)	2	2	23	54	58	1	60	58	2
Baltic Countries and Russia									
Estonia (3)	4	4	20	18	31	21	42	57	9
Latvia (3)	5	3	18	15	19	32	25	41	20
Lithuania (3)	3	3	21	–	–	–	42	57	8
Russia (4)	5	6	12	17	28	22	29	39	17
Eastern Europe									
Czech Republic (2)	3	2	22	26	32	14	29	37	18
Hungary (3)	7	9	8	19	34	19	26	47	16
Poland (3)	9	8	7	10	29	25	23	40	23
Ukraine (3)	–	–	–	19	29	20	45	61	6

continued

Central Europe

Austria (1)	4	6	17	33	36	10	35	38	15
Belgium (Flemish) (1)	8	6	11	34	45	8	26	37	22
Belgium (French) (1)	–	–	–	22	36	15	24	32	26
Netherlands (1)	–	–	–	47	56	3	22	35	25
Germany(e) (1)	6	6	14	33	46	7	34	44	12
Switzerland (1)	17	13	2	27	40	12	27	39	19
Southern Europe									
Croatia (3)	15	–	–	25	36	13	21	38	24
France (1)	4	12	4	11	23	31	15	23	33
Greece (2)	–	4	20	18	38	18	17	23	31
Italy (1)	–	–	–	28	48	9	17	23	32
Malta (1)	–	–	–	40	56	4	18	25	30
Portugal (1)	12	5	6	11	21	34	19	26	29
Slovenia (3)	–	–	–	26	42	11	34	44	13
Spain (1)	–	–	–	25	32	16	26	25	28
TFYR Macedonia	–	–	–	11	26	27	6	17	35
North America									
Canada (2)	8	8	10	23	34	17	41	44	10
USA (2)	13	12	5	11	21	33	23	30	27
Israel (2)	38	22	1	13	· 25	28	11	21	34

Notes:
(a) Source: Rehm *et al.*, 2004: 1023–6.
(b) Abstention is defined as reporting never having had a drink.
(c) Source: Gabhainn and François, 2000: 104.
(d) Source: Schmid and Gabhainn, 2004: 75, 80.
(e) Figures are from selected cities and do not represent the entire country.

cent of those aged 16–21 in a Zambian sample reported using alcohol in the last 12 months, while the figures for 15–21 year-olds in two locations in South Africa were 73 per cent and 90 per cent (Nkowane *et al.*, 2004). Surveys of Namibians aged 12–16 found only 13 per cent of girls and 23 per cent of boys drinking at all prior to independence in 1990, although the percentages increased thereafter (see Jernigan, 2001: 16; Skjelmerud, 2003: 621). A qualitative study of drinking among Namibian young women found that drinking, and indeed heavy drinking, had a number of meanings for them: as an expression of equality and solidarity, but also on the other hand as a marker of social class and distinction; as a way of forgetting and a time out, but on the other hand as a metaphor for power and an expression of protest (Skjelmerud, 2003). Non-drinkers, in contrast, often saw abstinence as associated with ambition, as a choice between 'getting drunk and getting somewhere'.

Hazardous patterns of consumption

In addition to abstinence and age of initiation into drinking, drinking patterns differ substantially from country to country. An important aspect of drinking patterns, in terms of the health and social hazards from drinking, is the extent to which consumption is concentrated in heavy drinking occasions. As part of the World Health Organization's Global Burden of Disease analysis, a hazardous drinking score was developed on the basis of survey data and expert judgements, to characterize the degree of hazard associated with each litre of alcohol in a given country (Rehm *et al.*, 2004). Along with drinking in public places and not with meals, the score gives primary weight to the extent to which heavy drinking occasions predominate in the drinking culture in the country. The third column of figures in Table 8.1 shows the population-weighted average hazardous drinking score for the 14 WHO global sub-regions. Regions with the most hazardous drinking patterns are Russia, South-East Asia, Eastern Europe and parts of Africa. Western European countries, particularly those in the wine region, and Japan and Australasia in the Western Pacific tend to display the least hazardous patterns of drinking.

The Hazardous Drinking Score refers to drinking patterns among adults. While no such score is available globally for youth populations, in many societies young people's alcohol consumption is at a more hazardous level than that of the corresponding adult population (Windle, 1999). Adolescents and young adults tend to drink more per occasion and drink to intoxication in a higher percentage of their drinking occasions, when compared with adults. It is precisely the 'prized but dangerous' psychoactive effects, as Steele and Josephs term them, of drinking heavily that are sought by youth (Room, 2003; Steele and Josephs, 1990). This will be discussed more in the next section of this chapter.

A common argument in the USA suggests that US drinking customs would be improved and harms reduced if children were taught to drink at the family table, as had traditionally occurred in France (Heath, 1995). While French young people drink more often than those in the USA, US youth are more likely to have been drunk by the age of 15 (see Table 8.2). Table 8.2 shows the hazardous drinking score (Rehm *et al.*, 2004) for countries participating in the 2001/2002 Health Behaviour in School-Aged Children (HSBC) Study (Schmid and Gabhainn, 2004). It is clear that young people in similarly patterned countries can and do show somewhat divergent patterns of drinking. For example, of the pattern 3 (more hazardous drinking) countries, the ratio of intoxication to drinking occasions is higher for youth in the Nordic countries (Iceland 0.88, Finland 0.83, Greenland 0.73, Sweden 0.62, Norway 0.61) as opposed to Eastern Europe (Ukraine 0.66, Latvia 0.39, Estonia 0.38, Poland 0.36, Russia 0.29). This indicates that while young people in both of these areas are likely to drink to intoxication, they are more likely to do it on most of their drinking occasions in the Nordic countries. In fact, young people in the Eastern countries, with the exception of Ukraine, show ratios of intoxication to drinking occasions that are more like those seen in pattern 2 countries than those seen in other pattern 3 countries. Finally, young people in pattern 1 countries drink to intoxication far less frequently, and with a lower intoxication/drinking occasion ratio than other countries (Portugal 0.22, France 0.15, Italy 0.15, Malta 0.11, Cyprus 0.06), in line with the drinking style of the adults in these countries.

However, news reports suggest that young people's drinking patterns are becoming more similar across countries – young people in the wine regions of Europe are drinking more in the fashion of North American and Nordic drinking styles, leading to a more homogeneous drinking culture among youth (Biagorri, Fernández and GIESyT, 2004; Donato *et al.*, 1995; Hibell *et al.*, 2000; Weill and Le Bourhis, 1994). This is in part attributed to a rise in the club culture, with the 15–24 age group being more than ten times more likely than the general population to be frequent club visitors (Chatterton and Hollands, 2003). Globalization and internationalization of youth cultures have resulted in a move away from nationally based youth cultures to a more global and eclectic mix of music locales and behaviours (Carrington and Wilson, 2002). Across Europe and North America, the consumption locales are merging, while societies have become less authoritarian and marriage occurs later in life (Kiernan and Eldridge, 1987). As this homogenization is occurring, the general trends, which have been noted in the USA by the Monitoring the Future (MTF) study, and in Europe in the HBSC studies and the ESPAD study, have been for rates of heavy episodic drinking and drunkenness to rise (Gabhainn and François, 2000; Hibell *et al.*, 2000; Johnston, O'Malley and Bachman 2002a). Comparing across the survey years in the late 1990s, in over one-third of the countries the level of drunkenness has increased, and in only one has it decreased.

Similar trends seem to have occurred in developing nations. Traditional societies were often heavily age- and gender-graded, with access to alcohol reserved for older males. Today, as they become emancipated, young people, including younger well-educated women, are drinking more often and more heavily (Jernigan, 2001; Room *et al.*, 2002; Suggs, 1996).

The role of alcohol in coming of age

In the developed world, the average age of those who have consumed at least one glass of wine, beer or other form of alcohol is about age 13 (Schmid and Gabhainn, 2004). Initiation of drinking thus happens at the beginning of a transition into young adulthood and is a time of changing roles, responsibilities and lifestyles. While drinking may occur somewhat later among the majority of surveyed youth in developing and Asian countries, there are population sub-groups who begin at much earlier ages (Day, 1998; Haworth and Acuda, 1998; Isaac, 1998; Rocha-Silva, de Miranda and Erasmus, 1995; Yucun and Zuxin, 1998).

In modern developed societies, and to a lesser extent in the developing world, the child is protected from joining the adult world too early. It is the responsibility of adult society (parents, teachers, etc.) to prepare the child for entry into adulthood, and often laws exist to prevent children from entering adult roles too early. In particular, with respect to alcohol there are age minimums for drinking and penalties for breaking these. The 'social clock' is a concept used by sociologists to refer to the time when behaviours are appropriate to be taken on. For example, in the developed world holding a full-time job is as inappropriate for a 12 year-old as is not holding one by the age of 25 (Neugarten, Moore and Lowe, 1965; Room, 2003). However, youth is a time of learning to take on new roles and can be a period of experimentation. During this time, young people undergo change in virtually every domain of life; they are completing their education, entering the workforce, finding partners, and perhaps getting married and starting families. During this period of emancipation, young people often act ahead of the normative standards that are set out for them, and thus without adult supervision and within a complex and fluid social environment. During this time, risk-taking tends to increase, especially in terms of a number of health-risk behaviours (Galambos and Leadbetter, 2000). Increasingly, research suggests that a primary reason that young adults experience more risk-taking behaviour is that they are exploring their identities and are not yet restrained by roles of increased responsibility such as parenthood or work (Arnett, 1998, 2000). The transition from the role of child to young person to adult is highly governed by cultural expectations. These expectations can differ between cultures, and the type of experimentation and the degree to which it occurs and is accepted also differ between cultures (for more detail on the cultural variation in the coming of age process see Room (2003)).

The level of acceptance of youth drinking prior to the official drinking age is quite inconsistent across cultures. In traditional wine regions, drinking often begins early and consists initially of wine with family meals, and drunkenness is in principle discouraged (Beccaria, 2002); whereas in regions such as the USA and northern Europe, daily consumption is not sanctioned, alcohol consumption is discouraged as long as possible, and, as we have seen, a greater proportion of drinking occasions involve drinking to drunkenness. On the other hand, banalizing drinking in wine-drinking cultures does not necessarily prevent youthful intoxication. A recent qualitative study of Parisian young people, mostly in their early 20s, found that the largest group drank only on weekends, often to intoxication, and rejected drinking daily or drinking red wine as associated with 'alcoholism' (Freyssinet-Dominjon and Wagner, 2003).

Drinking alcohol is but one of many new behaviours included in this period of emancipation (Gusfield, 1996). Driving a car, getting a job and having sex are some of the more accepted behaviours that are expected of most people as they progress into adulthood; however there are also other actions, such as drinking early in youth, trying drugs, vandalism and violence that are not expected behaviour within the main part of society (Room, 2003). But whether the behaviours are expected or not, the social clock is set so that they are expected to start, if at all, typically during the same life-stage. Risk behaviours thus are often initiated at about the same age. They often also occur within the same physical context for young people; underage drinking and sex, for example, are both more likely to occur when parents are absent and youth are gathering together. Young adults also are not necessarily skilled in handling difficulties and challenges that arise while they are negotiating their way through these new behaviours. For example, they have less experience of driving than adults and thus tend to experience motor vehicle accidents at lower blood alcohol concentrations (BAC) than adults (McLean, 1983). Also, inexperienced young people are typically less secure in their sexuality than adults, and thus the negotiation of a sexual situation with a potential new partner is more likely to result in unexpected and undesired outcomes (Beale, Dusseldorp and Maes, 2001; Long, 1976).

The initiation of these different behaviours at around the same age means that they often occur in conjunction. But the conjunction may be situational or coincidental, rather than necessarily showing that one behaviour is causing another. Indications that increased alcohol consumption and other high-risk behaviours are life-course related is backed up by the finding that these behaviours tend to decrease as people enter marriage and take on other new roles of increased responsibility (Arnett, 2000; Stephen and Squires, 2003).

Youth drinking and intoxication in hazardous events

The three leading forms of mortality among young people – accidental death, homicide and suicide – are associated with alcohol use (Hingson and Kenkel, 2003; World Health Organization, 2000). Part of the relation is due to the effects of drinking, and particularly of intoxication, on physical co-ordination. Drunkenness universally affects such actions as co-ordination and the ability to reason, and with a large enough amount of alcohol in the system, physical incapacity results. As a result of this physical incapacity, we can see increased accidents and victimization amongst those who drink larger quantities.

Another part of the relation between drinking and such behaviours as aggression or risky sexuality is more variable and culturally mediated. Experiments (mostly conducted among US college students) find that drunkenness increases aggressive acts (Lang, 1983; Taylor, 1993), and (although more equivocally) sexual acting-out (Bullock, 2001; Woods and Mansfield, 1983). While neurophysiological connections are important, cultural and personal beliefs also play an important role in these connections (Graham, West and Wells, 2000; MacAndrew and Edgerton, 1969). In many cultures, there is a strong belief that intoxication causes aggression, including sexual aggression, and also a strong belief that it causes sexual acting-out. These beliefs are conventionally referred to in terms of 'disinhibition'.

Often, expectations about the disinhibitory effects of alcohol are somewhat gender-specified. Stereotypically in many cultures for males intoxication is associated particularly with violence while for females cultural expectations and concerns revolve around sexual acting-out. Thus, among younger adults in Ontario, males were more likely than females (22 per cent vs. 15 per cent) to think it was likely they themselves would become aggressive and possibly violent if they had 'a few drinks, enough to feel the effects' (Ferris, Templeton and Wong, 1994: 21). In a US experimental study of interactions between an unacquainted dyad (woman and man), drinking alcohol increased both the man's and the woman's perception that each was behaving more sexually and in a more disinhibited way. The alcohol effect was greater on the men's perceptions, which the authors interpret in terms of 'society's negative messages regarding women's alcohol consumption and sexuality' and 'women's vulnerability to sexual and non-sexual aggression when intoxicated' (Abbey, Zawacki and McAuslan, 2000: 689).

It is clear that alcohol-related changes to social comportment are not consistent across cultures (MacAndrew and Edgerton, 1969; Room, 2001). Changes for the worse in behaviour that violate norms – behaviour that is defined as illegal, immoral, unethical or sinful – are highly dependent upon culture and cultural norms. Thus there is cultural variation in whether people act more violently when drinking or in the extent to which they become more sexual after drinking.

The belief in the connection of intoxication with sexual actions and with aggression thus has consequences. It has been shown that alcohol expectancies are well formed in children by the age of 12, and that these expectancies can predict – to an extent – their levels of alcohol consumption, and to a lesser extent their behaviour while intoxicated (Dunn and Goldman, 1996). In effect, young people holding more positive expectancies towards alcohol tend to drink more often, and in larger quantities, than those who have more negative expectancies (Jones, Corbin and Fromme, 2001). Ultimately, as a young person gains more experience drinking and obtains feedback regarding the accuracy of pre-existing expectancies, they are modified, and then predict future drinking patterns to an even higher degree (Leigh and Stacey, 2004). Taking this analysis one step further, it can be shown that people's expectancies regarding alcohol's effects upon their sexual behaviour can act like a self-fulfilling prophecy (George et al., 2000; Leigh, 1990).

Further, expectancies related to intoxication can become an excuse for behaviour that is otherwise difficult to justify to others, or to oneself (Bullock, 2001; Scott and Lyman, 1968; Scully and Marola, 1984). Getting into fights, having sex with someone who you would not want to see again (or even be seen with), acting too rowdily or damaging someone else's belongings are all often blamed on intoxication, when one is drinking. Such excuses are self-serving, and used often in an attempt to reduce the individual's responsibility in the event. These excuses can act to reduce the negative effect (guilt or shame) associated with an action or to avoid damaging one's identity, or to avoid punishments or sanctions that otherwise might result. That 'everyone knows' that intoxication causes bad behaviour diminishes the value of the excuse, inviting the question, if the drinker knew that, why did he or she get intoxicated? The benefit of the excuse is thus more likely to occur for those who are younger, and more inexperienced. Once one is older and 'should' know better, the value of alcohol as an excuse may decrease (Room, 2001).

Societies generally recognize that popular views about the excuse value of intoxication can offer a defence of the otherwise indefensible, so in most legal systems the general principle is that intoxication is not an excuse (Sheehy, 1996). At the level of publicly expressed opinions, for instance in population surveys on attitudes in North America and Sweden, most young people also agree that intoxication is no excuse. More privately, for instance in discussions in focus groups, young people in Sweden agree that intoxication is in fact used informally as an excuse, and that to a certain degree it 'works' in lessening the blame for, or merely normalizes or justifies the occurrence of a particular 'bad' behaviour (Tryggvesson 2004).

The role of intoxication as an excuse is seen in particular with first-time sexual encounters with a new partner. Young adults often use alcohol both as an explanation of why the sex occurred, and of why sexual protection was not used. Wide agreement in a culture that intoxication is disinhibiting may, on the other hand, result in special precautions when a risky situation is foreseeable. While event-level analyses show that young adults who are drinking are more likely to engage in sex, the analyses have consistently shown that drinking is unrelated to condom use (Bullock, 2001; Leigh, 2002). One way of understanding these findings is that to the extent that intoxication is expected to produce more risk-taking, young people do exercise forethought about their nights out and potential sexual encounters. What otherwise might be an effect of intoxication is counteracted by the planning ahead or by the rules people make for themselves about what to do, and not to do, when intoxicated. Disinhibition turns out to be something that may often be reflexive and subject to forethought, rather than an automatic response in the moment.

Alcohol-related expectancies explain a moderate portion of the variance in how much young adults drink, and in how they behave when drinking. However, the recognition of their role has raised the issue of whether behaviour can be changed or risk forestalled by changing expectancies. The accomplishment of this could then help to reduce some of the harmful consequences that youth experience with heavy drinking. Efforts to change alcohol expectancies are essentially efforts to change the cultural beliefs about the effects of intoxication. While the literature on this for college students offers some hope, at this point the support is extremely limited (Jones, Corbin and Fromme, 2001; Wiers et al., 2003). Programmes designed to change expectancies have resulted in short-term changes in the drinking patterns primarily of men; however, there is little change in those of women. Further, there is even less support for the idea that changes in drinking patterns are mediated via changes in expectancies (Dunn, Lau and Cruz, 2000; Wiers et al., 2003). Long-term effects are virtually untested, with some of the longest experimental studies looking at success only three months after the expectancy challenge (Dunn, Lau and Cruz, 2000). However, this line of research is still in its infancy and may yet prove successful in providing some long-term change for the better in the drinking patterns of young people and the harmful effects – accident, injury, homicide and suicide – that can result from them.

Conclusions

Young people's drinking in a given society generally reflects adult drinking in quantities and patterns. Much of what we know of consumption and alcohol-related problems comes from the developed world where surveys have been more systematic and inclusive. Data from the developing world are often based on the more westernized segments of the population.

Lifelong abstention rates differ around the world by gender, religion and region; with women and Islamic areas reporting higher rates of abstention, and with lower rates located in the wine regions of the world. Although these rates do go down with age, the contrasts seen between cultures and by gender do remain throughout adulthood.

Overall, where it has been measured, young people's alcohol consumption has been on the rise over the past 30 to 35 years, with the exception of a brief downturn in the late 1980s and early 1990s. Rates of consumption and drunkenness are currently on the rise again, around the world. The gender gap is beginning to decrease; young women's rates of abstention are decreasing, and rates of drunkenness are increasing. However, young men are still more likely to drink regularly and to become drunk than are young women.

Drinking to intoxication is not equally prevalent in different regions of the world. In developing countries, among those who do drink, it is quite common to drink to intoxication. Of the developed countries, youth in the Nordic countries and in Britain are the most likely to drink to intoxication, followed by youth in the Baltic countries and elsewhere in Eastern Europe. Drinking patterns are, however, becoming more similar across countries, reflecting trends also seen in adults. This homogenization also probably results from the globalization of youth culture, that has young from many countries dancing to the same music, wearing similar clothes, and watching the same movies. This homogenization is bringing with it increasing levels of intoxication.

Drinking begins at transition into adulthood in many cultures, which is often earlier than adults would like. This occurs as a multiplicity of risks are being faced and young people are exploring new identities. Heavy drinking, alcohol-related problems and associated risky and illegal behaviours all peak during late adolescence and early adulthood, particularly in the developed nations. The role that alcohol plays in this stage is particularly ruled by cultural expectancies.

While alcohol universally has effects upon co-ordination and the ability to reason, cultural and personal beliefs also play an important role in defining the consequences of intoxication, such as aggression and sexual activity. Expectancies about the disinhibitory effects of alcohol are related to the amount of alcohol consumed and the consequences experienced.

In the past, efforts at increased taxation (resulting in higher prices for alcoholic beverages) and increasing the minimum age for drinking have been the most successful mechanisms in reducing underage drinking (Babor *et al.*, 2003). However, altering culturally based attitudes and expectancies may provide a future direction to reduce both alcohol consumption and the harms associated with it, since there are limits to how high the drinking age can be raised and how much tax a country will agree to charge.

References

Abbey, A., Zawacki, T. and McAuslan, P. (2000) 'Alcohol's effects on sexual perception', *Journal of Studies on Alcohol*, 61: 688–97.

Arnett, J.J. (1998) 'Risk behavior and family role transitions during the twenties', *Journal of Youth and Adolescence*, 27: 301–20.

Arnett, J.J. (2000) 'Emerging adulthood: A theory of development from the late teens through the twenties', *American Psychologist*, 55: 469–80.

Babor, T., Caetano, R., Casswell, S., Edwards, G., Giesbrecht, N., Graham, K., Grube, J., Gruenwald, P., Hill, L., Holder, H., Homel, R., Österberg, E., Rehm, J., Room, R. and Rossow, I. (2003) *Alcohol – No Ordinary Commodity: Research and Public Policy*, New York: Oxford University Press.

Beale, J., Dusseldorp, E. and Maes, S. (2001) 'Condom use self-efficacy: Effect on intended and actual condom use in adolescents', *Journal of Adolescent Health*, 28: 421–31.

Beccaria, F. (2002) 'Young people in a wet culture: Functions and patterns of drinking', *Contemporary Drug Problems*, 29: 305–34.

Biagorri, A., Fernández, R. and GIESyT (2004) *Botellón: Un Conflicto postmoderno [Botellón: A Postmodern Conflict]*, Barcelona: Icaria.

Bonnie, R.J. and O'Connell, M.E. (2004) *Reducing Underage Drinking: A Collective Responsibility*, Washington, DC: The National Academies Press.

Bullock, S.L. (2001) *About Last Night: Dates, Drinks and Sex. A Study of the Association Between Alcohol Use and Sexual Activity Among Heterosexuals, Including Sexual Behaviour at High Risk for the Transmission of STDs and HIV*, Unpublished Dissertation, University of Toronto, Toronto.

Carrington, B. and Wilson, B. (2002) 'Global clubcultures: Cultural flows and late modern dance music culture', in M. Cieslik and G. Pollock (eds) *Young People in Risk Society* (pp. 74–99), Aldershot: Ashgate.

Chatterton, P. and Hollands, R. (2003) *Urban Nightscapes: Youth Cultures, Pleasure Spaces and Corporate Power*, London: Routledge.

Day, J. (1998) 'Southeast Asia', in M. Grant (ed.), *Alcohol and Emerging Markets: Patterns, Problems and Responses* (pp. 107–22), Ann Arbor, MI: Brunner/Mazel, Taylor Francis Group.

Donato, F., Monarca, S., Chiesa, R., Feretti, D., Modolo, M.A. and Nardi, G. (1995) 'Patterns and covariates of alcohol drinking among high school students in 10 towns in Italy: A cross-sectional study', *Drug and Alcohol Dependence*, 37: 59–69.

Dunn, M.E. and Goldman, M.S. (1996) 'Empirical modelling of an alcohol expectancy memory network in elementary school children as a function of grade', *Experimental and Clinical Psychopharmacology*, 4: 209–17.

Dunn, M.E., Lau, H.C. and Cruz, I.Y. (2000) 'Changes in activation of alcohol expectancies in memory in relation to alcohol use after participation in an expectancy challenge program', *Experimental and Clinical Psychopharmacology*, 8: 566–75.

Ferris, J., Templeton, L. and Wong, S. (1994) *Alcohol, Tobacco and Marijuana: Use, Norms, Problems and Policy Attitudes among Ontario Adults* (Research Document No. 118), Toronto: Addiction Research Foundation.

Freyssinet-Dominjon, J. and Wagner, A.C. (2003) *L'alcool en Fête: Manières de Boire* de la Nouvelle Jeunesse Étudiante [Alcohol as a Party: Ways of Drinking of the New Student Youth], Paris: L'Harmattan.

Gabhainn, S.N. and François, Y. (2000) 'Substance use', in C. Currie, K. Hurrelmann, W. Settertobulte, R. Smith and J. Todd (eds), Health and Health Behaviour Among Young People (pp. 97–114), Copenhagen, Denmark: World Health Organization, European Office.

Galambos, N.L. and Leadbetter, B.J. (2000) 'Trends in adolescent research for the new millennium', International Journal of Behavioural Development, 24: 289–94.

George, W.H., Stoner, S.A., Norris, J., Lopez, P.A. and Lehman, G.L. (2000) 'Alcohol expectancies and sexuality: A self-fulfilling prophecy analysis of perceptions and behaviour', Journal of Studies on Alcohol, 61: 168–76.

Graham, K., West, P. and Wells, S. (2000) 'Evaluating theories of alcohol-related aggression using observations of young adults in bars', Addiction, 95: 847–63.

Gusfield, J. (1996) Contested Meanings: The Construction of Alcohol Problems, Madison: University of Wisconsin Press.

Haworth, A. and Acuda, S.W. (1998) 'Sub-Saharan Africa', in M. Grant (ed.), Alcohol and Emerging Markets: Patterns, Problems and Responses (pp. 19–90), Ann Arbor, MI: Brunner/Mazel, Taylor Francis Group.

Heath, D.B. (1995) 'An anthropological view of alcohol and culture in international perspective', in D.B. Heath (ed.), International Handbook on Alcohol and Culture (pp. 328–47), Westport, CT: Greenwood Press.

Hibell, B., Andersson, B., Ahlström, S., Balakireva, O., Bjarnasson, T., Kokkevi, A., and Morgan, M. (2000) The 1999 ESPAD Report: Alcohol and Other Drug Use Among Students in 30 European Countries, Stockholm, Sweden: CAN (The Swedish Council for Information on Alcohol and Other Drugs).

Hingson, R. and Kenkel, D. (2003) 'Social, health and economic consequences of underage drinking (Background paper)', in R.J. Bonnie and M.E. O'Connell (eds), Reducing Underage Drinking: A Collective Responsibility (pp. 351–82), Washington, DC: The National Academies Press.

Isaac, M. (1998) 'India', in M. Grant (ed.), Alcohol and Emerging Markets: Patterns, Problems and Responses (pp. 145–76), Ann Arbor, MI: Brunner/Mazel, Taylor Francis Group.

Jernigan, D.H. (2001) Global Status Report: Alcohol and Young People (Vol. WHO/ MSB/MSB/01.1). Geneva: Substance Abuse Department, Department of Social Change and Mental Health, World Health Organization.

Johnston, L.D., O'Malley, P.M. and Bachman, J.G. (1991) Drug Use Among American High School Seniors, College Students and Young Adults, 1975–1990 (Vol. 1: DHHS Publication No. ADM 91-1813), Washington, DC: Government Printing Office.

Johnston, L.D., O'Malley, P.M. and Bachman, J.G. (2002a) Monitoring the Future: National Survey Results on Drug Use, 1975–2001 (Vol. 1: Secondary School Students (NIH Publication No. 02-5106)), Bethesda, MD: National Institutes on Drug Abuse.

Johnston, L.D., O'Malley, P.M. and Bachman, J.G. (2002b) Monitoring the Future: National Survey Results on Drug Use, 1975–2001 (Vol. 2: College Students and Adults Ages 19–40 (NIH Publication No. 02-5107)), Bethesda, MD: National Institutes on Drug Abuse.

Jones, B.T., Corbin, W. and Fromme, K. (2001) 'A review of expectancy theory and alcohol consumption', *Addiction, 96: 57–72*.

Kiernan, K.E. and Eldridge, S.M. (1987) 'Age at marriage: Inter and intra cohort variation', *The British Journal of Sociology*, 38: 44–65.

Lang, A.R. (1983) 'Drinking and disinhibition: Contributions from psychological research', in R. Room and G. Collins (eds), *Alcohol and Disinhibition: Nature and Meaning of the Link* (DHHS Publication No. (ADM) 83-1246), pp. 48–99, Rockville, MD: National Institute for Alcohol Abuse and Alcoholism.

Leigh, B.C. (1990) 'The relationship of sex-related alcohol expectancies to alcohol consumption and sexual behavior', *British Journal of Addiction*, 85: 919–28.

Leigh, B.C. (2002) 'Alcohol and condom use: A meta-analysis of event-level studies', *Sexually Transmitted Diseases*, 29: 576–482.

Leigh, B.C. and Stacey, A.W. (2004) 'Alcohol expectancies and drinking in different age groups', *Addiction*, 99: 215–27.

Long, I. (1976) 'Human sexuality and ageing', *Social Casework*, 57: 237–44.

MacAndrew, C. and Edgerton, R.B. (1969) *Drunken Comportment: A Social Explanation*, Chicago: Aldine Publishing Company.

McLean, A.J. (1983) 'Alcohol, drugs and road accidents', *Medical Journal of Australia*, 1: 596–7.

Neugarten, B.L., Moore, J.W. and Lowe, J.C. (1965) 'Age norms, age constraints, and adult socialization', *American Journal of Sociology*, 40: 710–17.

Nkowane, B.L., Rocha-Silva, L., Saxena, S., Mbatia, J., Ndubani, P. and Weir-Smith, G. (2004) 'Psychoactive substance use among young people: Findings of a multi-centre study in three African countries', *Contemporary Drug Problems*, 31: 329–56.

Rehm, J., Room, R., Monteiro, M., Gmel, G., Graham, K., Rehn, N., Sempos, C.T., Frick, U. and Jernigan, D. (2004) 'Alcohol', in M. Ezzati, A.D. Lopez, A. Rodgers and C.J.L. Murray (eds), *Comparative Quantification of Health Risks: Global and Regional Burden of Disease Due to Selected Major Risk Factors* (Vol. 1, pp. 959–1108), Geneva, Switzerland: World Health Organization.

Rocha-Silva, L., de Miranda, S. and Erasmus, R. (1995) *Alcohol, Drug Use and Related Matters: Young Black South Africans (10–21 years)*, Pretoria: Centre for Alcohol and Drug Research, Human Sciences Research Council.

Room, R. (2001) 'Intoxication and bad behaviour: Understanding cultural differences in the link', *Social Science and Medicine*, 53: 189–98.

Room, R. (2003) 'Drinking and coming of age in a cross-cultural perspective (Background paper)', in R.J. Bonnie and M.E. O'Connell (eds), *Reducing Underage Drinking: A Collective Responsibility* (pp. 654–77), Washington, DC: The National Academies Press.

Room, R., Jernigan, D., Carlini-Marlatt, B., Gureje, O., Mäkelä, K., Marshall, M., Medin-Mora, M.E., Monteiro, M., Parry, C., Partanen, J., Riley, L. and Saxena, S. (2002) *Alcohol in Developing Societies: A Public Health Approach* (Vol. 46), Helsinki: Finnish Foundation for Alcohol Studies, in collaboration with the World Health Organization.

Schmid, H. and Gabhainn, S.N. (2004) 'Alcohol use', in C. Currie, C. Roberts, A. Morgan, R. Smith, W. Settertobulte, O. Samdal and V.B. Rasmussen (eds), *Young People's Health in Context: Health Behaviour in School Aged Children (HBSC)*

Study: International Report from the 2001/2002 Survey (No. 4 ed., pp. 73–83), Copenhagen, Denmark: World Health Organization.

Scott, M.B. and Lyman, S.M. (1968) 'Accounts', *American Sociological Review*, 33: 46–52.

Scully, D. and Marola, J. (1984) 'Convicted rapists' vocabulary of motive: Excuses and justifications', *Social Problems*, 31: 530–44.

Sheehy, E. (1996) 'The intoxication defense in Canada: Why women should care', *Contemporary Drug Problems*, 23: 595–630.

Skjelmerud, A. (2003) 'Drinking and life: The meanings of alcohol for young Namibian women', *Contemporary Drug Problems*, 30: 619–45.

Steele, C.M. and Josephs, R.A. (1990) 'Alcohol myopia: Its prized and dangerous effects', *American Psychologist*, 45: 921–33.

Stephen, D.E. and Squires, P.A. (2003) '"Adults don't realize how sheltered they are." A contribution to the debate on youth transitions from some voices in the margins', *Journal of Youth Studies*, 6: 145–64.

Suggs, D.N. (1996) 'Mosadi tshwene: The construction of gender and the consumption of alcohol in Botswana', *American Ethnologist*, 23: 597–610.

Taylor, S.P. (1993) 'Experimental investigation of alcohol-induced aggression in humans', *Alcohol Health and Research World*, 17: 108–12.

Tryggvesson, K. (2004) 'The ambiguous excuse: Attributing violence to intoxication – Young Swedes about the excuse value of alcohol', *Contemporary Drug Problems*, 31: 231–61.

Weill, L. and Le Bourhis, B. (1994) 'Factors predictive of alcohol consumption in a representative sample of French male teenagers: A five-year prospective study', *Alcohol and Drug Dependence*, 35: 45–50.

Wheeler, R.H. and Cunter, B.G. (1987) 'Change in spouse age difference at marriage: A challenge to traditional family sex roles', *The Sociological Quarterly*, 28: 411–21.

Wiers, R.W., Wood, M.D., Darkes, J., Corbin, W.R. and Sher, K.J. (2003) 'Changing expectancies: Cognitive mechanisms and context effects', *Alcoholism: Clinical and Experimental Research*, 27: 186–97.

Windle, M. (1999) *Alcohol Use Among Adolescents* (Vol. 42), London: Sage.

Woods, S.C. and Mansfield, J.G. (1983) 'Ethanol and disinhibition: Physiological and behavioral links', in R. Room and G. Collins (eds), *Alcohol and Disinhibition: Nature and Meaning of the Link* (Vol. DHHS Publication No. (ADM) 83-1246, pp. 4–26), Rockville, MD: National Institute for Alcohol Abuse and Alcoholism.

World Health Organization (2000) *International Guide for Monitoring Alcohol Consumption and Related Harm*, Geneva: World Health Organization: Department of Mental Health and Substance Dependence.

Yucun, S. and Zuxin, W. (1998) 'China', in M. Grant (ed.), *Alcohol and Emerging Markets: Patterns, Problems and Responses* (pp. 123–44), Ann Arbor, MI: Brunner/Mazel: Taylor Francis Group.

Part III

Special circumstances, special needs?

special needs?

Chapter 9

Sex, drugs and vulnerability

Young people who sell sex and use drugs

Cheryl Overs and Chris Castle

Despite a range of national and international laws and policies intended to prevent it, children and young adults continue to be involved in selling and trading sex in most parts of the world. In some places, it even appears that younger people may have become more involved in sex work since the HIV epidemic began, as a result of men seeking younger sexual partners in the belief that they are more likely to be HIV negative (PANOS/UNAIDS 2000).

Drug taking also is a worldwide phenomenon among young people from various backgrounds, and generates vulnerability to HIV and AIDS in various ways, depending on the drug and the setting (see chapters 6 and 7). Added to this, the trend towards migration to swelling urban centres is accelerating in many places, resulting in conditions such as large slums, very high unemployment and a breakdown of supportive social structures that open the way to increases in young people's involvement in commercial sex and drug use.

This chapter explores some of the issues raised when children and young adults are involved in the sex trade and drugs. It looks primarily at vulnerability to HIV, while stressing that marginalized young people often face a mix of circumstances that drive a mix of vulnerability that includes violence, premature pregnancy, overdose, discrimination and various other physical and mental problems that are not discrete from each other nor separable for the purposes of programme planning and policy. It points to the need for greater conceptual clarity and stronger multi-sectoral approaches to enable the integration of services that address the various vulnerabilities identified.

Young people and commercial sex: bringing the picture into focus

Discussions about young people and commercial sex are invariably characterized by definitional fogginess, primarily about the meaning of terms such as 'young' and 'commercial sex', but also about the meanings of consent, payment, work, exploitation and abuse. There is universal consensus that all efforts should be made to prevent prepubescent children selling or trading sex, or working in the sex industry at all because of the associated risks of mental and physical trauma, and a range of other ethical, religious and normative values.

Children under the local age of consent are being abused where adults are having sex with them, paid or unpaid, and in such a situation the best option is that which ends the abuse. In places with well-developed social support for children and effective non-corrupt law enforcement, this will mean involvement and contact with the relevant authorities. Unfortunately, this is not a viable strategy in many countries where no support is available, or worse, where authorities themselves are complicit or engaged in drugs and commercial sexual abuse (Busza, Castle and Diarra 2004).

Because the potential for these vulnerabilities does not stop at puberty, young people in their early teens who are selling or trading sex are often viewed as subjects of sexual abuse in the same way as younger children. But working with young people in their mid-teens presents some of the most difficult practical and ethical issues for programme planners and health and social workers in the field. Understanding the issues around young people selling sex so as to develop appropriate responses is not helped by the influence of international agencies and agreements that define childhood as the period before reaching the age of 18.

Significantly, local laws set the age at which people can legally consent to sex, often at 16. Combining pre-pubescent children and young men and women as old as 17 together masks their very different circumstances and provides little guidance on the ethical issues around sexuality and sexual exploitation and abuse. This is especially problematic in places where economic independence and reproductive life often begin soon after puberty, especially in very poor communities. Here, people who have reached puberty but who are not yet 18 years old will be young adults, and many will be legally entitled to enter into sexual relations.

Selling sex, trading sex

Around the world, for many school-age children who survive alone and homeless or in poor conditions, daily life is a mix of legal and illegal income and resource generating activities and social life, including sex for pleasure and income. Many of these activities generate risk in one way or another, together with externally determined labels. Different labels tend to be ascribed by different types of agencies depending on their interests or mandates. Agencies that provide services such as accommodation and welfare are likely to label them as homeless, with the young people being called street kids, pavement dwellers, and so on. Drug services and law enforcement agencies may categorize the same individuals as drug dependents or users and/or criminals, while HIV/AIDS and STI service providers may view these same young people as sex workers.

This process of labelling young people can restrict the development of more holistic, or integrated, responses to the overarching factors that contribute to vulnerability related to sex and drugs. Because AIDS agencies are concerned with sexual behaviour, young people who sell sex are often labelled as victims of sexual abuse or as prostitutes. Where young people trade sex for resources and in-kind payments rather than cash or sell sex intermittently, they are often dubbed informal sex workers (UNAIDS 2002).

These labels are unlikely to capture the multiple roles of a young person living in a poor community who, within a 24 hour period, may be a school child, a carer looking after his/her younger siblings, a street vendor helping his/her parent, a sex worker, a child playing with friends (Ball and Howard 1995). Community and service provider perceptions differ according to the context within which they are in contact with the young person (e.g. in school, during street outreach, at a health service, or when being detained by police). As a result, different needs and risks are defined, which in turn results in different, and often very narrow, responses.

Perhaps as unhelpful as confusion around these ethical issues is the tendency for many researchers, service providers and theoreticians to pathologize the sexuality and sexual behaviour of marginalized young people. Discourses around young people, sex and drugs are frequently limited to a model of dichotomous relationships in which victimhood and exploitation are posited against the notion of choice and ideas about the essential characteristics of healthy non-exploitative relationships.

However, as Grabosky has pointed out, from the perspective of the young person things may be quite different:

> Many children do not regard themselves as exploited. For some, the experience is part of the grim reality of life on the street. Some are seeking affection or a feeling of self-worth often unavailable from other sources. Others appreciate having a degree of autonomy, notwithstanding the very real constraints on their life choices.
>
> (Grabosky 1998: 39)

How drugs and commercial/transactional sex combine to create vulnerability

Legal and illegal drugs, both injected and non-injected are used throughout the world. There are well-documented patterns of drug use throughout the world and some less well known. Cannabis is the most commonly used illegal drug globally and alcohol is the most commonly used legal drug. In the Americas and the Caribbean, cocaine is common and it is injected, inhaled and smoked as crack. In the Commonwealth of Independent States and many other North Asian countries, opioids dominate and injecting is common, while in South and South East Asia, drug use is more varied, including opioids and, more recently, amphetamine-type stimulants.

Less well documented are patterns of drug use throughout Africa, although individual studies and recent media attention show that a variety of drugs are used including manufactured drugs such as methaqualone (Mandrax) as well as opioids, cocaine, and amphetamine-type stimulants (e.g. 'ecstasy'). A Nigerian drug agency recently reported that a 'large number of young people in Nigeria are using cannabis, alcohol, khat and inhalants and those who abuse drugs also engage in risky sexual behaviour, exposing themselves to diseases like AIDS and other sexually transmitted ailments' (Anti-Drug Agency 2004).

In many places where drug use has been presumed to be either low or confined primarily to older people and men, recent research reveals increases in drug use among young people, including women. This is the case in India, where young women are taking up opioids and amphetamines in significant numbers (Sankar 2004).

Solvent/inhalant abuse, commonly known as glue sniffing, has often been reported among homeless or marginalized children, and occurs in every continent (Voice of America News 2004).

Although there are some universal issues, the nature and extent of young people's involvement in drugs and prostitution vary between settings and individuals. The various drugs themselves, the context in which they are used and the way in which sex is exchanged for money or other resources all have a profound influence on risk taking and vulnerability to HIV. To develop effective policy and strategies we need to look at a broad range of sexual and drug taking behaviours.

The links between drug use, commercial sex and young people's vulnerability to HIV are not simple or amenable to generalization. When a person injects drugs, the risk of acquiring HIV can become extremely high and the risk of both acquisition and transmission may be further heightened where that person also sells or trades sex. This is not inevitable, however, and programmes to prevent HIV infection that reach sex workers who inject can be as successful as programmes working with other vulnerable populations. While some male, female and transgender sex workers also inject drugs, many injecting drug users (IDUs) exchange sex for money or drugs some time in their drug using careers. Furthermore, many IDUs buy sex from sex workers (MAP 2001; MAP 2004; UNDP 2004).

The contexts and constraints in these different life situations may be quite different. Gender, age and identity play major roles in defining these situations of risk, as do different drugs and different patterns of drug use. Young people often say they take drugs for fun, to enable them to stay alert longer, to relieve psychological and/or physical pain, to alleviate boredom, isolation and distress, or in the case of some drugs, notably solvents, to relieve hunger.

Injecting clearly carries the most direct risk of HIV transmission if injecting equipment is reused among different drug users. It is crucial, however, not to overlook the other ways in which drugs fuel sexual risk taking and vulnerability. One way is where regular and dependent drug users' need for drugs causes them to sell unprotected sex or exchange it for drugs (UNESCAP 2003).

A third way in which the risk of HIV transmission can be heightened derives from the manner in which drugs and alcohol can break down inhibitions. Like other drug users and drinkers, sex workers and their clients may be more likely to have unprotected sex as a result of intoxicating effects that reduce the ability to control situations, make appropriate decisions and practise safer sex. This applies to a broad range of intoxicating substances, including alcohol, and it applies to those who buy sex as well as those who sell it.

Reducing harm and vulnerability: whose responsibility?

The relative merits of various actions aimed at reducing vulnerability among young people who sell sex and use drugs is a contentious subject. This is at least partly because harm reduction strategies such as providing condoms and syringes can be seen as colluding with or encouraging drug taking and the commercial abuse of children and/or young people.

In reality, difficult decisions, often at individual or case level, have to be made about how to work with young adults generally and those taking drugs or selling sex in particular. Here, the imperative is often seen as prevention of HIV, hence the focus on immediate harm reduction measures, with additional support and services to follow when possible. Where the main drugs are opioids and injecting is the main method used, harm reduction services that include drug substitution therapy, needle and syringe supply, HIV treatment and drug education and rehabilitation services orientated towards youth are crucial to help young women and men to avoid acquiring or transmitting HIV.

Where there is a clear overlap between drugs and formal sex work, it is possible to implement integrated services that address both. Recently, in Eastern Europe and the Commonwealth of Independent States, the Open Society Institute and International Harm Reduction Development have begun supporting agencies that reach female sex workers to incorporate harm reduction into their work (Simon 2001). In the Islamic Republic of Iran, community-based Triangular Clinics are being expanded throughout the country to provide integrated prevention and management of HIV/AIDS, drug use/dependence, sexually transmitted infections and hepatitis. These clinics are also linked with similar services in the Iranian prison system to ensure continuity of care and follow up for those entering or leaving prison (WHO/EMRO 2004).

While adults often associate peer influence with so called risky or deviant choices, social networks and peers can also play an important 'protective' role. Successful projects may be those that build on networks and increase their beneficial aspects and reduce their negative potential using what can be called a 'youth-centred' approach. Local programmes have identified innovative ways of reaching vulnerable young people, who, despite their very difficult lives, and perhaps because of them, often respond well to certain services and environments. Shelter, food, warmth, food and escape from abusive older people have all worked well to attract young people into non-judgemental services in various countries (Shaw and Aggleton 2002).

Improved and multi-disciplinary understandings of the dynamics of vulnerability can lead to stronger programmes and better interventions. We need to understand more about the transition from exchanging sex informally to working in the formal sex industry. Several factors combine to influence not only why some young people take drugs and sell or trade sex, but how vulnerable they are when they are doing it. We can both understand and respond to that vulnerability better by viewing sex and drug taking through a 'socio-ecological perspective' that considers environmental factors such as poverty, social isolation, cultural norms, gender roles, family, school and peers, as well as individual factors such as cognitive maturity, self-efficacy and sexual knowledge.

Policy and the law

Health and social welfare interventions provided by government and NGOs are rarely likely to attain the quality and coverage needed to reduce the vulnerability of young people in most developing countries. This means that the laws and policies that govern responses to drug taking and prostitution are particularly important. Some have been particularly controversial. Recently, a war on drugs in Thailand attracted criticism for violence against drug users and widespread violations of human rights (Human Rights Watch 2004). It also appears to have been largely ineffective, leading to a change in stated government policy by the time of the 2004 Bangkok International AIDS Conference.

Similarly, sex industry raids by police, authorities and some NGOs that ostensibly aim to liberate children have resulted in violence, destruction of property and subsequent homelessness of many of the poorest women and their families in India, Cambodia and Bangladesh among others (Empower 2002).[1] Even where raids do not violate the human rights of sex workers,

---

1 For more information, and to access discussions about the impact of 'rescues' and brothel closures, see the Network of Sex Work Projects website at www.nswp.org or http:// archives.healthdev.net/sex-work

rescuing child prostitutes is often not a straightforward solution. The success of any kind of 'rescue' depends to a large degree on the alternative provided. Children repatriated to abusive families or inadequate institutions will remain vulnerable and other alternatives need to be sought (UNIFEM/ UNIAP 2002).

Policy development should be informed by the perspective of young people who live and earn money to survive in dangerous conditions who often describe the ways in which their situation is worsened by stigma, discrimination, violent institutions and social alienation. The following quotations from Brazilian street kids illustrate some of the discriminatory attitudes and roles the police, authorities and the public can play in perpetuating abuse and vulnerability. In this respect, it is salutary to note that the first young woman speaks about escaping to rather than from the streets, and decides to sell sex to reduce her vulnerability to violence.

> I started living on the street when I was seven years old, when I lost my mother and couldn't survive. Me and my brother were hungry and then a friend of mine took me to the street and I became a prostitute. Then I started to steal because as a prostitute I couldn't support my family. When I started thieving the men came to arrest me, they beat me up and did a lot of things. They put me in jail . . . and then I was taken to FEBEM (The Foundation for Child Welfare) and beaten again. I used to spend one or two months in prison and then I would escape to the street again. I used to take drugs and start stealing again, and then get arrested and beaten up. Always stealing and getting beaten up. When I got fed up with being beaten I went back to being a prostitute but then the bastards slap me around if I don't want to have sex with them.
>
> (Dimenstein 1991: 23)

> We sniff glue to forget our hunger. It changes our minds and makes us forget tons of things. Like discrimination. We can't get on a bus because people think we are going to steal.
>
> (Dimenstein 1991: 3)

There are clear signs in Brazil of policy change having resulted in improved conditions since the mid-1980s, when an estimated half a million young women and girl children under the age of 18 were selling sex (Dimenstein 1991: 5), and estimates of numbers of children living on the streets reached eight million (Dimenstein 1991: 2).

Policies and interventions that change public perceptions and reduce discrimination against vulnerable young people include ensuring that police and welfare and justice institutions behave lawfully and sympathetically and prosecute those who abuse children rather than the children. In Brazil, these changes are at least partly due to advocacy and awareness raising nationally and internationally by human rights organizations and the many NGOs set up to work with young people living on the streets in the wake of the well-publicized carnage of street children by death squads.

There has also been a particularly promising civil society response to child prostitution in India, that has led to a quantifiable decrease in underage sex workers in one area. Adult sex workers in Calcutta have formed a self-regulation board to regulate the influx of newcomers to the area (UNESCAP 2003). Women they judge as being too young to work in the sex industry are not permitted to work, and appropriate arrangements are made for them such as alternative employment, placing them in residential educational facilities and arranging for sensitive repatriation, depending on the circumstances. For the adult sex workers in the association, this is not only a human rights issue in respect of the young women, they hope that it will help reduce violent raids in the name of rescuing underage girls from sex work by police, state powers and NGOs. Engaging communities of adult sex workers in reducing child prostitution by responding appropriately on an individual case basis could be developed further as a model.

Another important model is to offer short-term or emergency support services that provide shelter and immediate assistance to young people especially in need: for example, very young girls and boys, those who are ill and in need of urgent medical attention, and those in especially dangerous circumstances. These kinds of actions and interventions are sometimes described as being 'low threshold', because their entry criteria are more easily met than longer-term services. The aim is for them to provide a bridge to longer-term support and services. Temporary shelter is different from a drop-in centre that typically does not provide residential facilities, but can offer a 'one-stop shop' of services to minimize the need for service users to travel to several different service points in pursuit of assistance. Critical within this range of service provision is the priority of supporting access to good quality education, right for all people regardless of circumstances. A good quality education considers the needs of the learner, and in the instance of young people using drugs and selling sex, creative and innovative learning opportunities may be called for as an alternative to school-based learning that may not correspond to the needs of these young people.

Interventions for young people in crisis situations, such as living on the street, homeless, involved in drug cultures, street cultures and/or prostitution, can also provide an important entry point to services. Again, a holistic approach is critical to address the most pressing immediate needs (which might be for shelter, medicines, treatment for drug abuse or food) whilst incorporating harm reduction efforts and working towards getting the young person to a place of safety, and relationships of trust and confidentiality. Only when the crisis is over, longer-term welfare and health needs are met and new skills, confidence and resources are in place can damaged young people begin leading safe and productive lifestyles (O'Neil, Green and Mulroy 1997).

The often multiple and complex needs of young people involved in commercial sex and drug use can overwhelm service providers struggling to ensure the availability of a holistic range of support including education, access to housing, food and nutritional support, medical care, social justice and inheritance rights. Yet there are plenty of examples where inability or unwillingness to connect young people to all these services will foil attempts to improve their quality of life. The lessons from decades of development work have clearly taught us that there is no point in preventing people from suffering or dying as the result of a specific disease or social problem, if something else will do it instead.

As important as it is to provide a comprehensive range of services responding to the needs of the population, the attitudes, awareness, sensitivity and skills of service providers are also vitally important. Just because young people involved in commercial sex and drug use may appear more difficult to reach and work with than other types of young people, this does not abrogate the need to involve, respect and listen to them. Young people from all backgrounds, social classes and circumstances will remind service providers, if given the chance, that youth are not a homogenous group. Organizations providing services must remember that beyond the numerous labels of sex worker, drug user, street kid, lie young individuals with specific needs and aspirations. No one appreciates being lumped into a group, with their needs generalized and left unmet.

Many young people who sell sex and use drugs are marginalized, perhaps violent and often difficult to work with. Some governments, faith-based organizations and others may refuse to work with them or attach conditions about sobriety and sexual abstinence that effectively prohibit access for many young people who need the service. This may be a result of moral views or fear that non-judgemental services in some way condone the behaviours of the group. Some organizations, health workers and NGO staff involved in HIV prevention, care, treatment and support may not see these young people as falling within their mandate, but youth associations and others working with young people may not either. If some services are extended to young people selling sex and using drugs, are these properly tailored and specific to their needs? How do we realistically organize a comprehensive and appropriate range of services, with what actors, which correspond to the needs of the young people concerned, and what from their perspective are the key questions?

This is where the rationale for a multi-sectoral approach becomes clear. However, practical examples of where such an approach functions well remain disappointingly scarce. Those who work with vulnerable young people know very well that no matter how obvious and important collaboration with others may be in theory, there are a number of well-known barriers to achieving it in practice. Where a range of different service providers do succeed in coming together to provide a spectrum of necessary services for young people involved in commercial sex and drug use, the common ingredients for success are often a functioning mechanism to facilitate good communication and understanding such as local consortia or networks, donors that understand and support a collaborative approach among distinct service providers, linkages between government and civil society, and leadership among the service providers characterized by an openness to collaboration and co-ordination.

Often overlooked, but very much at the centre of any working multi-sectoral approach, is the meaningful involvement of the community or group targeted, with their needs, interests and perspectives taking prominence in the planning and delivery of services. Involving young people in service planning and delivery who may come from experiences of commercial sex and drug use may pose considerable challenges to some providers. However if an organization is not capable of learning how to meaningfully involve young people, it is probably also not capable of providing appropriate and effective services worthy of donor and community support.

A way forward

Throughout this chapter, we have alluded to the need for policy reform that brings definitions of youth close to a reality that service providers and young people can recognize. We have also stressed the importance of understanding and valuing the role that can be played by adults working in commercial sex, alongside sex workers' rights to respond to child sexual abuse and young people's involvement in prostitution. Effective policies and strategies are those that take account of a broad range of sexual and drug taking behaviours, the contexts in which these occur, and how gender, age, poverty, culture and identity play important roles in defining situations of risk.

The importance of multi-sectoral approaches to effectively reach young people and respond to their needs is vital, but must be underpinned by respecting young people themselves and the essential contribution they can (and must) make to addressing the vulnerabilities they face. National authorities and service providers must find ways of overcoming overly compartmentalized programmes, as well as those that fail to link up in a way that delivers comprehensive and easily accessed services with the service user firmly at the centre. Successful approaches may be those that build on existing social networks, enhancing the beneficial elements that can result from positive peer influence and support, while seeking to reduce the possible negative peer behaviours that can result in greater vulnerability.

Policies and legislation are more likely to change for the better when the perspectives of young people are articulated and acted upon as part of overall advocacy efforts, linked when possible to national and international human rights campaigns. Advocacy by NGOs working with young people on the streets will resonate more forcefully when carried out collectively and coherently.

Harm reduction strategies, as with other well-intentioned interventions, need to be adjusted to the setting and context in order to be effective, such as addressing specific drug using contexts (e.g. ensuring ready access to sterile needles and syringes where drugs are injected, providing sexual risk reduction education to crack cocaine users, educating pharmacists about the needs of drug users wanting to purchase injecting equipment). The adaptation of the strategies can occur more easily when the young people affected are at the centre of the response, and when service providers and local workers orient themselves to this critical necessity.

References

Anti-Drug Agency (2004) 'Plea to Teachers and Parents', *East African Standard*, 22 June.

Ball, A. and Howard, J. (1995) 'Psychoactive substance use among street children', in T. Harpham (ed.) *Mental Health and Urbanization in Developing Countries*, Aldershot: Avebury.

Busza, J., Castle, S. and Diarra, A. (2004) 'Trafficking and health', *British Medical Journal*, 328: 1369–71.

Dimenstein, G. (1991) *Brazil: War on Children*, London: Latin America Bureau.

Empower (2002) *Rescues in Thailand: Human Rights Violations. A report on the human rights violations women are subjected to when 'rescued' by anti-trafficking groups who employ methods using deception, force and coercion*, Chiang Mai: Empower.

Grabosky, P. (1998) *The Commercial Sexual Exploitation of Children: A Stocktake and Analysis for Australia's National Action Plan*, Canberra: Australian Institute of Criminology.

Human Rights Watch (2004) *Not Enough Graves: The War on Drugs, HIV/AIDS, and Violations of Human Rights in Thailand*. Online. Available HTTP: http://www.hrw.org/campaigns/aids/2004/thai.htm (accessed 19 August 2004).

MAP (2001) *The Status and Trends of HIV/AIDS/STI Epidemics in Asia and the Pacific*, Melbourne: MAP.

MAP (2004) *AIDS in Asia: Face the Facts*, Bangkok, Thailand: MAP. Online. Available HTTP: http://www.mapnetwork.org/reports.shtml

O'Neil, M., Green, J. and Mulroy, S. (1997) 'Young people and prostitution from a youth service perspective', in D. Barrett (ed.) *Child Prostitution*, London: The Children's Society.

PANOS/UNAIDS (2000) *Informing the Response to HIV*, Nov. 2000. Online. Available HTTP: http://216.239.59.104/search?q=cache:nYDi6E0dwv4J:www.panos.org.uk/files/menandhivinzambia.pdf+%22Informing+the+response+to+HIV%22+%2BZambiaandhl=en

Sankar, A. (2004) 'Women Start Early', *The Hindu Times*, 26 June.

Shaw, C. and Aggleton, P. (2002) *Preventing HIV/AIDS and Promoting Sexual Health Among Especially Vulnerable Young People*, Faculty of Social Sciences,

University of Southampton, Southampton: Safe Passages to Adulthood Programme/DFID/WHO.

Simon, S. (2001) 'Linking sex workers with harm reduction', *Newsletter of the International Harm Reduction Development Program and the Open Society Institute*, Spring 2001, 2: 10–12.

UNAIDS (2002) *Sex Work and HIV/AIDS, UNAIDS Technical Update* (Geneva: UNAIDS). Online. Available HTTP: http://www.unaids.org/html/pub/publications /irc-pub02/jc705-sexwork-tu_en_pdf.htm

UNDP (2004) *Reversing the Epidemic: Facts and Policy Options*, Bratislava: UNDP.

UNESCAP (2003) *HIV/AIDS Prevention Care and Support: Stories from the Community*, Bangkok: United Nations Economic and Social Commission for Asia and the Pacific.

UNIFEM/UNIAP (2002) *Trafficking in Persons: A Gender and Rights Perspective*, Bangkok, Thailand: UNIFEM. Online. Available HTTP: http://www.unifem-eseasia.org/resources/others/traffic.htm

Voice of America News (2004) *UN Annual World Drug Report*, 25 June.

WHO/EMRO (2004) *Best Practice in HIV/AIDS Prevention and Care for Injecting Drug Abusers: The Triangular Clinic in Kermanshah, Islamic Republic of Iran*, Cairo: WHO. Online. Available HTTP: http://www.emro.who.int/ASD/ BackgroundDocuments/STD-052.pdf

Chapter 10

Young migrants, refugees and displaced people

Mary Haour-Knipe, Linda Eriksson and Danielle Grondin

Although migration has taken place for millennia, population movement has become both more frequent and more complex in recent years. Reasons for the increase in migration include social and economic imbalances between rich and poor countries, combined with increasingly available means of communication and of fast and simple transport.

The process of migration is often described as one marked by disruption, differences and difficulties. Migration may mean losing the support of families and friends, as well as familiar ways of life. Refugees and internally displaced people may have lost jobs, their possessions, family members and even their dignity. Migration is also marked by differences, for example of culture and of language, that may set the migrant apart from his or her neighbours.

Yet migration can also have positive effects: for the migrant, for whom successful migration may bring increased safety, improved economic well-being, and increased coping skills and mastery; for the receiving society with the arrival of a young and generally healthy new work force; and for the sending society in the form of remittances sent home by workers abroad, and new ways of thinking they bring home when they return.

After a brief review of the size and nature of migration globally, this chapter describes some of the challenges to health and development faced by young migrants. It focuses on young people who move voluntarily, as well as upon young people who may be displaced through war and civil conflict. It also considers the special circumstances and needs of unac-companied minors and young people who are trafficked. In keeping with the theme of this book, special attention is given to sexual health and substance use.

Size and nature of global migration

Currently, one in every 35 persons worldwide is an international migrant. Eighty-six million people migrated for reasons of work in 2003, of whom some 32 million are in developing countries (International Labour Organization 2004). The year 2003 saw some 17 million refugees and internally displaced persons, the vast majority of whom also remain within developing countries (UNHCR 2004). Partly as a result of tightening restrictions on immigration and on labour migration, recent years have also seen an increase in the numbers of persons smuggled and trafficked. The International Organization for Migration estimates that some 4 million persons were trafficked in 2002 (International Organization for Migration 2003).

The last ten years have seen an increased feminization of migration, with women currently representing about 50 per cent of the estimated 175 million migrants worldwide. In Asia, in particular, women now make up the majority of expatriates working abroad: accounting for 65 per cent of all Sri Lankan and 70 per cent of Philippino migrant workers overseas (International Organization for Migration 2003). A growing number of rural-to-urban migrants within developing countries are also young women, attracted by the increasing availability of factory and services jobs in large cities, including domestic service (Martin 2004). It is difficult to estimate how many migrants are young people, as available data does not separate youth from adults or children. We know, however, that some 43 per cent of the world's refugees and internally displaced persons are under the age of 18 (UNHCR 2004).

Young migrants, sex and substance use

Sexual attitudes and practices – and also attitudes towards drug use – are coloured by social expectations, and influenced by cultural norms and by religious beliefs. Norms and behaviours often shift when a young person is transposed from one place to another. Although many young people navigate such journeys very well, some may become confused, finding themselves vulnerable to exploitation by employers and by those who deal in the trafficking of drugs and of human beings.

Sexual behaviour and relationships are profoundly influenced by culture, and misunderstanding new situations by utilizing old conceptual frameworks can cause confusion. Young women and men who move from a conservative society to one perceived to be more liberal, in particular, may be ill equipped to deal with apparent sexual freedom. They may not understand the norms or the limits in the new society, or how to protect themselves.

Such factors can put young women at risk of undesired pregnancy, or of sexually transmitted infections, including HIV, in ways that are strikingly similar across cultures. Whether they are coming from Myanmar or Laos to work in factories in Thailand (Ford and Kittisuksathit 1996), from Portugal to Switzerland (Fontana and Beran 1995) or from rural to urban areas within South Africa in search of work (Pick and Cooper 1997), young migrant women from more conservative cultures may have received little education in sex and relationships, especially since sexuality is not talked about at home. No longer under the protection of family members in the new location, and not having developed the relational tools that guide safer behaviour in the host culture, some may be ill equipped to control their own behaviour and to deal with sexual negotiation.

Cultural misunderstandings may also cause difficulties for men. Shtarkshall and Soskolne (2000) describe how such problems can arise for Ethiopian and Russian immigrants in Israel for example. When they observe public physical contact between Israeli youth, some young immigrant men interpret the behaviour the way they would have at home, and assume that their Israeli counterparts are sexually active. And since the physical contact is not always limited to one person, they may assume that Israeli youth are 'promiscuous'. Having grown up in a culture in which sexual matters are regulated by strong external controls many such young men are unable to recognize the internalized personal controls in force among their counterparts in the new culture. This may lead some to make potentially serious mistakes in their approaches to young women, and others to feel alienated and estranged.

Across all continents, migrant women in transit have been found to be at risk of rape, and of transactional sex to continue a journey, or sex for survival. To give just one example, a study of transit stations in Central America showed that women are often forced to exchange sex in lieu of cash in order to cross borders. Undocumented migrants who have been deported, in particular, may lack economic resources and have little means of defending themselves against aggression. Transactional sex, survival sex and non-consensual sex may occur in conditions that place individuals at risk of infection with HIV and STIs since condom use is infrequent (Bronfman *et al.* 2002).

The Coordination of Action Research on AIDS and Mobility (CARAM) network has worked extensively with female migrant workers in Asia, especially restaurant, hotel and factory workers, entertainers, sex workers and domestic workers. Such women are vulnerable to violence, abuse, subordination and discrimination, especially in the unregulated informal sector. Domestic workers often have little education, coming from remote villages to urban centres, sometimes migrating to work as young as ages 15 or 16. Lack of protection and lack of access to appropriate services and information increases their vulnerabilities to exploitation and violence, and also compromises their health (Coordination of Action Research on AIDS and Mobility Asia 2002).

A study of young people in Tanzania has highlighted how increasing urbanization and intensification of rural poverty have been accompanied by an increase in the migration of young people from rural to urban areas. Many young migrants are ill equipped for gainful employment, and homelessness, sex work, street vending, and child labour were found to be commonplace. Questionnaires and in-depth group discussions were carried out with young Tanzanian in-migrants living on the streets in Dar es Salaam, many of whom were street vendors and/or involved in sex work. The young women interviewed lived in shared overcrowded rooms, the boys often slept in abandoned

vehicles, at bus stops and in bars. Substance use was frequent, with marijuana used to give confidence to endure difficult working conditions and lack
of food (Nantulya *et al.* 2001).

The same study also examined the conditions of young refugees in the
Mtabila refugee settlement in Kigoma, Western Tanzania. Most of the
refugees interviewed had no parents, and lived in family-like groups in
the camp. They reported that the major problems were related to sexuality, mental health, and uncertainty about their future. Some had become
informal sex workers. Rape was reported, the offenders fellow refugees and
men from neighbouring communities. Both boys and girls reported being
lonely and depressed, and fearing for their future (Nantulya *et al.* 2001).

Loneliness is an underestimated but potent risk factor that may encourage
people of any age to engage in behaviours that put them at risk of HIV and
other STIs, or of substance use, and young people who have immigrated
recently may be especially vulnerable. In a survey of 2,635 high school
students in Massachusetts in the USA, for example, those who had lived in
the country for six years or less (n = 191) were likely to report greater peer
pressure to engage in risk behaviours including use of tobacco, alcohol and
drugs, and engaging in sexual intercourse. They also reported less parental
support, and were less self-confident in their ability to refuse substance use
(Blake *et al.* 2001).

A number of studies, mainly carried out in developed countries, have
examined health behaviours and substance use among immigrant youth. In
a study of a representative sample of 9,300 15 to 20 year olds in Switzerland,
those who were children of labour migrants from southern or southeastern
European countries showed more, although subtle, difficulties than their
Swiss counterparts – including minor signs of depression, feeling they do not
get along with their parents, poorer body image. More of the immigrant than
of the Swiss boys reported having had more than five sexual partners, and
also slightly more lifetime use of cocaine and heroin (5 per cent versus 2 per
cent) (Ferron *et al.* 1997).

With respect to migration and substance use, a distinction should be
made between young people who use drugs when they are on the move, and
young migrants established in communities who use illicit drugs on a more
regular basis. An exploratory study among young female substance users of
Surinamese descent in the Netherlands sheds light on some of the factors
influencing substance use. Because of difficulties outsiders may encounter
entering the highly structured Dutch job market, some Surinamese immigrants may continue the 'free trade' street culture practised in Surinam. In
the Netherlands, this grey circuit is well suited for drug dealing, receiving
and other petty crimes. Many of the women interviewed reported that social
security benefits were not sufficient to cover their needs. As a result, they
sought extra income from sex work, and petty crimes such as shoplifting and
credit card fraud (van de Wijngaart 1997).

Numerous US studies have examined the evolution of substance use among young immigrants over time. Such studies show that with time both sexual and substance use behaviour among immigrants comes to resemble that of counterparts in the destination country. Initially, the children of immigrant families experience better health and adjustment than do children in US-born families. The picture deteriorates with time in the host country, however. In differences that remain after family income and other potentially confounding factors are controlled for, immigrant youth living in the USA for longer periods tend to be less healthy, and to report more risk behaviours such as early first sexual intercourse, delinquent or violent behaviour, and tobacco or other substance use (Hernandez and Charney 1998).

Several other recent US studies reveal a similar trend. As they become more adapted to the new culture, Hispanic girls in the USA engage in sexual activity at earlier ages, are more likely to give birth outside marriage, and to leave school. Spanish speaking young people who consider themselves highly acculturated to US society report increased use of alcohol, tobacco and drugs (Brindis *et al.* 1995). Among Massachusetts high school students (Blake *et al.* 2001) and among boys attending middle schools in Florida (Vega *et al.* 2003) US-born young people and those who had lived in the country longer were significantly more likely than recent immigrants to use alcohol or marijuana, and to start illicit drug use earlier. Two large-scale national surveys, similarly, confirm the findings. Foreign-born young people have lower rates of substance use than those who are US-born, but risk behaviours increase as young people acculturate (Johnson *et al.* 2002, Gfroerer and Tan 2003).

Several hypotheses have been put forward to explain these findings. At the most immediate level, economic pressures to succeed, as well as the threat of deportation, may serve as powerful deterrents for recent immigrants to experiment with illicit substances, and/or to become dependent on legal substances (Johnson *et al.* 2002). In the longer term, it is probable that such differences are related to assimilation and integration into the host culture. The assimilation (or acculturation) model would posit that immigrants' substance use is a by-product of socialization into the host culture.

Alternatively, the stress of adjusting to a new environment may be lessened by substance use. Of particular importance are the social factors that exacerbate immigrants' stress. These include discrimination, poverty and restricted economic opportunities, poor quality housing (McKay *et al.* 2003), language barriers, cultural marginality, lack of access to health services (Verdurmen *et al.* 2004), family separation and other forms of social isolation and loss of social status.

Special circumstances, special needs

Internally displaced young people

All over the world, young people may be internally displaced within their own country as a result of famine, war, civil disturbance and other disasters. In countries where there are ongoing civil wars, the consequences can be both complex and dramatic as the Montería case study illustrates.

Forced internal displacement in the city of Montería

Five decades of internal conflict in Colombia have forced approximately 2 million people into internal displacement. Most of them are women and children under the age of 18. In contexts such as these – poverty, tensions between internally displaced persons and the host communities, family disintegration, labour exploitation and limited access to health and education – the vulnerability of young people to substance use and STIs may increase. To date, however, little hard research and few programmatic interventions have been carried out.

As part of a pilot project designed to address this gap, and also to explore the feasibility of efforts to reduce the vulnerability of internally displaced young people to STIs including HIV, a survey was carried out in 2003 among 1,728 young people aged 10 to 24 in Montería, a city on the northern coast of Colombia receiving large numbers of internally displaced persons. About half of the respondents were natives of the city: 15 per cent had arrived more than six years previously, 15 per cent between three and six years previously and 12 per cent more recently.

Reflecting the break-up of families as a result of displacement, a substantial proportion of the internally displaced young people lived with their employer, with friends or with a partner, whereas the vast majority of the Montería natives of the same age lived with their families. Birth rates were somewhat higher among internally displaced young people than among their native counterparts (9 per cent versus 6 per cent), and a third of the internally displaced young people who desired a child reported that the primary reason was loneliness.

Conservative attitudes towards sexual behaviour were more frequent among recent arrivals: 20 per cent of those in Montería less than three years reported having had their first sexual experience with their wife or husband, as opposed to 12 per cent of the native residents. No significant differences between immigrants and natives were found for alcohol consumption or for other drug use except for cocaine: slightly more of those living in Montería between three and six years (4 per cent) said they had tried cocaine at least once, compared with 1 per cent of the more recent arrivals and 2.5 per cent of the local population. Only 76 per cent of the recent immigrants said they had heard of AIDS, but HIV/AIDS awareness rose with length of residence in Montería. Condom use was very low among all groups, but increased with duration of residence.

After the study had been finished, and to gather more in-depth material, one of the authors (LE) returned to Montería to interview some of the young women and men who had participated in the study. All were recent migrants who had been forcibly displaced from rural areas, mainly without their families: only one of the young people now lived with both parents.

The young people described feelings of loss: their studies had been interrupted, and they had had to adapt to a life in which something that had been permanent and taken for granted – their attachment to the land – had been removed. The familiar and the well known had suddenly been ruptured: experience had demonstrated that few things in life could be taken as certain.

They described life as being harder in Montería, where they were unknown and where they now had to look for other sources of income. They said that Montería provided more alternatives for education, health, food and employment, but at the same time people showed less solidarity: you need money or contacts to gain access to education and employment, and they had neither. Nor did they have any real friends in Montería. Being internally displaced was also a source of stigma: many of their peers in the new place assumed that the young internally displaced persons had belonged to an armed group, or that they would be violent as a result of the violence they had seen.

Young displaced people interviewed described behaviour in Montería, including sexual behaviour and drug use, as being more liberal and more outgoing than at home. The men said that the people they knew do not use condoms, and that they could protect themselves adequately by not having sex with a girl who they believe had an STI. Young people said they found drug use to be much higher in the city, possibly because it is less socially accepted to use drugs in their home villages. They also explained that at home the militia has an important influence repressing drug use.

Interviewees said that it is easy to buy drugs such as cocaine and *bazuco*[1] in the neighbourhoods, outside the schools or through their friends. Drug use was more common among boys than among girls, one reason for the difference being that it is less socially accepted for a girl to use drugs. Male interviewees added that boys think they will be considered better lovers if they use drugs. But drugs also 'help you forget your problems'.

(Adapted from Erikson *et al.* 2004)

Much research on refugees and internally displaced persons (IDPs) has been carried out in developed countries. However, a recent review summarizes interviews with 3,000 young people and adults in three less developed conflict-affected regions: Kosovo, the north of Uganda and Sierra Leone (Women's Commission for Refugee Women and Children 2004). In each region, young people reported experiencing lack of parental care, social disconnection or marginalization, recruitment into local militia, gender-based violence and discrimination, parenthood, and exposure to STIs including HIV.

Those displaced by conflict may have been exposed to rape as a weapon of war (Donovan 2003). Other forms of sexual violence include sexual slavery and abuse, sexual exploitation, forced marriage and domestic violence. Young women are the principal targets of gender-based violence, which can have long-term psychological and social impacts. Women and children who have been raped, and especially those who become pregnant, fear rejection by their families and communities and the possibility that they may never be able to marry (Women's Commission for Refugee Women and Children 2004). Boys and men in camps are also vulnerable to sexual violence (Nduna and Goodyear 1997) although discussion of the subject is limited by strong taboos (Women's Commission for Refugee Women and Children 2004).

Young people in Kosovo, Uganda and Sierra Leone interviewed by Women's Commission researchers said that substance use increased during and after war. Young people of both sexes said they turned to drugs to forget the pain of the war (Women's Commission for Refugee Women and Children 2004). Displacement may also expose young refugees and IDPs to new drug using practices and norms. During the Afghan conflict, for example, refugees fled to camps in Iran and Pakistan where there was significant use of opium and heroin, including injection drug use. Some reports have also described heroin use among young refugee women, a behaviour previously unreported

---

1 A local drug preparation made of coca paste often mixed with leftovers of other drugs such as marijuana. This inexpensive drug is used mainly in low-income groups.

in Afghanistan (United Nations Office for the Coordination of Humanitarian Affairs 2004).

There is reason for concern about the long-term consequences of such changes. In a study carried out in 2001 in a region on the Pakistan–Afghanistan border, for example, extremely low levels of HIV awareness and high HIV risk behaviours were found among drug users, among whom Afghanis were especially vulnerable (Zafar *et al.* 2003). With the repatriation of over 3 million refugees back to Afghanistan, newly acquired drug using behaviours can be expected to follow at least some of them.

Refugee camp environments – independently of the country in which they are located – profoundly change gender, age and class relations, giving rise to the gender violence and the substance use already described (Turner 1999, Harrell-Bond 2000). Not infrequently, refugee camps offer an overcrowded environment in which everyone is restricted in their freedom of movement, dependent on external aid for housing and food, and unable to farm or otherwise engage in productive employment. Households are often single-parent or child-headed as a result of the conflicts that caused the camps to be created in the first place. Enforced idleness can contribute to loss of self-esteem resulting in anxiety and depression, substance use, domestic violence and family breakdown (Harrell-Bond 2000).

In these kinds of contexts, desperation, impoverishment, powerlessness and monotony facilitate the development of substance use problems (Johnson 1996). Refugee camps may also become sites for drug trafficking and dealing, with drug trafficking networks taking advantage of underemployed and often desperate refugees who have been waiting for resettlement for several years. Such was reported in the resettlement camps for Vietnamese refugees in Hong Kong (Hong Kong Special Administrative Region 2000). One of the consequences was the development of heroin use among a large percentage of the young refugees, who later then found it extremely difficult to find recipient countries willing to offer refuge (Nemayechi and Taveaux 1997).

Unaccompanied minors

Every year, several thousand young people around the world migrate unaccompanied. Just over 2,000 unaccompanied minors requested asylum in Belgium in 1999. The figure reached almost 5,000 in the Netherlands in the first nine months of 2000. And in Germany the number of unaccompanied minors has risen during the last 15 years from an estimated 5,000 to 10,000 per year (International Organization for Migration (IOM) 2001). Many, such as those coming to Italy from the Balkans at the turn of the twenty-first century, are driven by conflict, or by the death, disappearance or imprisonment of family members (International Organization for Migration 2001, Women's Commission for Refugee Women and Children 2004).

In other cases, such as unaccompanied migration to Thailand from Myanmar, parents or relatives may send their children abroad to escape from poverty, inadequate education or limited political freedom, or from human rights abuses or religious and political persecution (Physicians for Human Rights 2004). Some parents encourage young people to migrate alone, seeing this as a form of sustenance for the family. Other children are smuggled to join a family member living as an irregular migrant in the destination country.

Human Rights Watch (2002) has estimated that at least 1,500 unaccompanied children are present in Spain at any given time. Many come from poor neighbourhoods in Morocco, and have left school early with few job skills. In interview, they said they saw no future for themselves in Morocco and some had paid smugglers to help them travel to Europe. Some had made the move with the express or indirect encouragement of their families, and many reported being the only sources of support for their families. Others said they were fleeing broken or abusive homes.

A study for the International Organization for Migration (2001) has further explored the motivations and conditions under which young people may migrate alone to countries such as Belgium, Germany, Italy and the Netherlands from places as diverse as Romania, Ukraine, Nigeria, China, Afghanistan and Sri Lanka. Most set off filled with a sense of adventure, with little awareness of any danger involved. Some are lured by promises of better job opportunities, better income and sometimes marriage to someone from a 'wealthy' country.

Both of the above studies document wretched conditions for many such young people in transit or destination countries, including police abuse, detention in unsafe and unhygienic centres, not being given adequate medical care, extortion and theft and physical abuse by larger and older children.

Trafficked young people

A lucrative industry has developed in the trafficking of human beings for sexual exploitation. UNICEF (United Nations Children's Fund 2001) estimates that about 1 million children are forced into the sex trade every year throughout the world. In some countries, there is increasing demand for young women and girls, driven partly by the presumption that young persons are less likely to be infected with HIV (Willis and Levy 2002, UNDP 2003). Trafficking for sex work occurs on all continents. In Africa, recent reports have identified Lesotho, Mozambique, Malawi and a number of refugee-producing countries as key source countries for women and children trafficked to South Africa, with Malawian women also having been trafficked to European destinations. In addition, women from Thailand, China and Russia are being trafficked to Southern Africa (Martens *et al.* 2003).

In Asia, Physicians for Human Rights has documented the way in which hill tribe women in Thailand may find themselves vulnerable to trafficking and other forms of exploitation because of restrictions on level of educational attainment and confinement to the boundaries of their home district. Unless they migrate, such women may be effectively limited to employment either as hired farm labourers or as sex workers. Members of families who have lost their land to government projects are also forced to migrate to find work, something that is very difficult to do safely. Without full citizenship they are dependent on, and often at the mercy of, their employers (Physicians for Human Rights 2004).

Beyrer (2001) has written extensively about trafficking for sex work in southeast Asia, with a particular focus upon the experience of Shan women trafficked from Myanmar. Although abduction happens, as does outright sale of daughters among the poorest of the poor, trafficking usually starts with a job offer. The girl may be offered work as a waitress, a domestic, or in manual labour. Her family usually receives some money as an advance payment. This advance is charged against future labour, as are the bribes required to cross borders during travel to destination countries. On arrival the trafficker hands the girl over to a brothel agent. If she refuses to work, she is raped or beaten, often both. At destination, wages are further deducted for room and board, clothes and makeup, sometimes for condoms, antibiotics to treat STIs and for contraception. It may take up to a thousand or more sex acts to pay off debts, and many women are unable to do this.

Trafficking for sex work has also been documented in the countries of the European Union. Girls in Albania and in post-conflict Kosovo, for example, have been at risk of trafficking for sexual purposes (Women's Commission for Refugee Women and Children 2004), and there are indications that unaccompanied or separated children and young people from Central and Eastern Europe and the Balkans are being trafficked to different European countries for forced sex work (IOM 2001). Zimmerman *et al.* (2003) have studied the health risks and consequences of trafficking for young people. Interviews with 107 key informants and 28 trafficked young people showed that most had left home in order to earn money. All but one reported having been tricked by bogus employment opportunities. Risks to health included dangerous travel conditions during the course of being smuggled (for example travelling long distances while hidden in cramped spaces in cars) and, for half of the women, violence and sexual abuse. The women reported forced and coerced use of drugs and alcohol; societal restrictions and manipulation; economic exploitation, debt bondage and legal insecurity; and abusive living and working conditions. Health problems included injuries and illnesses from physical and sexual abuse; forced sex and sexual assault; and – not surprisingly – mental health symptoms such as tiredness, crying, headaches, sadness, and feeling tense.

Beyond survival – matters of resilience

We have so far stressed the negative and potentially risky aspects of migration for young people, and the factors that increase vulnerability. However, migration can also have a positive impact on young people in terms of mental health as well as in improvements in the general quality of life. Overcoming the challenges of migration can lead to feelings of increased mastery and teach adaptive skills: having had to cope with a variety of adjustments and difficulties, a young person may be better equipped to deal with the next set of challenges (Haour-Knipe 2001). To return to the themes of this chapter, a young person who has learned to cope and to adapt is apt to be better equipped to negotiate safe and satisfying sexual relationships, and less vulnerable to problems with drugs.

Several of the studies discussed above raise the question of resilience. Some young people who have undergone extremely traumatic experiences may nevertheless do surprisingly well. Turner (1999: 9) has argued that if refugee camp life is difficult for young men, some may 'grab hold of the liberating aspects of liminality rather than being paralysed by its disintegrating side': using the opportunity to find other ways to survive, finding unique opportunities to create new roles and to develop new expertise and skills that they may eventually take back home. As the Women's Commission for Refugee Women and Children (2004: 25) has put it:

> The impact of these experiences on young people varied greatly. Many died: others were abused in conflict and also committed abuses against others. [. . .] Many young people, however, also developed strong survival skills, which formed the basis of their ability to develop important life and coping skills once they returned to civilian life. Many achieved a sense of power and identity, which brought them self-esteem, confidence and a vision for creating better lives for themselves.

More generally, the literature suggests that 'bicultural' immigrants who are able to adapt to their new social environment while retaining important elements of their native culture, are less likely than others to develop health problems including substance use habits. Those who feel equally at ease in two cultures are more likely to be better adjusted in a new society: they may maintain the strengths of their home culture, but they also retain supportive social links to it, while at the same time developing the language and social skills needed to successfully negotiate their new cultural setting (Hernandez and Charney 1998).

Meeting young people's needs

Young migrants and refugees have many of the same needs for health and other services as other young people. These include health promotion and help for drug-related problems. Access to services is often difficult however. Hindrances can include language barriers, lack of information and of trust, and services that are culturally inappropriate. Providing services to the most vulnerable poses particular challenges. For example, it may be difficult for health care workers to recognize sexual abuse among migrant young people from cultures in which young women are protected through strict family codes. In such instances, issues that are traditionally taboo, such as incest and rape, may well go unmentioned in an attempt to safeguard the family's honour.

All young people need to be cared for by health care providers who are sensitive to their specific circumstances and needs. Young migrants, in addition, need access to service providers who have additional skills in cultural sensitivity and in interpersonal communication. Such skills can be provided through specialist training. Service providers who lack them may discourage clients, and inadvertently fail to respect traditional practices that are important to them. In the worst of cases, they may trigger situations of discrimination, insensitivity and intolerance. Two examples of successful programmes to promote the health of young migrants are given in the case studies.

Would-be labour migrants in South Africa

Being a country richer than its neighbours, South Africa attracts many young migrants in search of work. Not all find employment, and many live on the margins of South African society, subject to xenophobia and discrimination. HIV prevention messages do not always reach such young migrants, because of language problems and also because of problems of access to public health facilities. Attitudes towards sexuality in their home countries are often more conservative, and migrants' perceptions of South African openness may cause them to believe that people in the latter country are 'crude' and offensive. Soccer has been used to promote AIDS knowledge, awareness and skills among such young migrants. Written information and condoms were distributed during matches, but more importantly peer educators were trained, and young migrants were given the means by which they could get in contact with a local NGO working in AIDS-related issues.

(Cowan 2001)

Working with refugees

A number of programmes bring health promotion to refugees in camps throughout Africa, Asia and Europe. Their work includes making health services more young person friendly. In Karago, a camp for Burundian refugees in Tanzania, young people had hitherto been reluctant to share reproductive health facilities with their parents. Parents were unhappy to learn that their children – especially their girls – were sexually active, and young people were embarrassed and sensitive about the lack of privacy and the possibility of lack of confidentiality. A youth centre for refugees was established, providing recreational services such as video, games, traditional dances, as well as a library and some vocational training. A year after the centre was established, it also started providing health education and distributing condoms.

(cited in Shaw and Aggleton 2002)

Conclusions

This chapter began by pointing out that migration has always been with us, and is increasingly common. We end by saying that the migration process brings opportunities but also more negative consequences of different kinds, with different consequences for young people's physical, mental and social health. These include heightened vulnerability for HIV and other STIs, substance use problems, alienation, social and behavioural problems and social exclusion that in turn results in even greater vulnerability.

Risk increasing factors include separation from partners, families, friends and communities resulting in loneliness and increased susceptibility to pressures to take risks; exposure and access to drugs; cross-cultural misunderstandings, for example when sexual mores are more liberal in the host community, and immigrants lack the knowledge and experience for dealing with them; feelings of being caught between two societies, and unable to relate comfortably to either of them; and broken dreams which can drive people to desperate measures and to violence.

Vulnerability enhancing factors include lack of access to housing, jobs, health and social services; marginalization, or lack of integration into the new culture which reduces opportunities; xenophobia, stigma and discrimination which create alienation; poverty which can drive risk behaviours; lack of power and of legal protection; and of course sexual violence. In general, the fewer the choices available before immigration the greater the subsequent vulnerability.

As we have seen, successful programmatic responses include the development and provision of services that are both youth friendly and migrant friendly. Positive policy responses are just as important. These include measures to ensure access to decent housing, schools, health and social services regardless of legal status; and to improve conditions so that people do not have to relocate against their will in the first place, or may do so with as much protection as possible.

As chapters elsewhere in this volume illustrate, a great deal of information currently exists about young people, drug use and sexual health. An increasing amount of information is also available on migration. But all too often, these bodies of knowledge remain separate: not enough research combines to focus simultaneously on migration, young people, and drug use and sexual health.

In ways that are only beginning to be understood, migration brings both risks and opportunities for young people and for societies. The risks are that young migrants will fall ill or become frustrated, turning their anger towards the societies they perceive as treating them unfairly. The opportunities lie in forging strength and resilience through coping and learning, and thus ultimately creating more resilient societies.

References

Beyrer, C. (2001) 'Shan women and girls and the sex industry in southeast Asia: political causes and human rights implications', *Social Science and Medicine*, 53: 543–50.

Blake, S.M., Ledsky, R., Goodenow, C. and O'Donnell, L. (2001) 'Recency of immigration, substance use, and sexual behavior among Massachusetts adolescents', *American Journal of Public Health*, 91: 794–8.

Brindis, C., Wolfe, A.L., McCarter, V., Ball, S., Starbuck-Morales, S. (1995) 'The associations between immigrant status and risk-behaviour patterns in Latino adolescents', *Journal of Adolescent Health*, 17: 99–105.

Bronfman, M., Leyva, R., Negroni, M. and Rueda, C. (2002) 'Mobile populations and HIV/AIDS in Central America and Mexico: research for action', *AIDS*, 16: S42–9.

Coordination of Action Research on AIDS and Mobility (CARAM) Asia (2002) Regional Summit on Foreign Migrant Domestic Workers. Online. Available HTTP: <http://caramasia.gn.apc.org/page.php?page=publications/reportsandtitle= CARAMASIA.ORG%20::%20Publications%20::%20Reports>.

Cowan, K. (2001) *Migrants from Africa Playing Soccer Against Aids: Final Report*, Pretoria: IOM.

Donovan, P. (2003) 'Rape and HIV/AIDS in Rwanda', *The Lancet*, 360: 17–18.

Erikson, L., and Guamizo, C., Mejia, A. and Prieto, F. (2004) *Jóvenes afectados por el desplazamiento en Montería frente a la salud sexual y reproductiva, las ITS y el VIH/Sida*, Organizacion International para las Migraciones, Bogota, DC, Colombia.

Ferron, C., Haour-Knipe, M., Tschumper, A., Narring, F. and Michaud, P.A. (1997) 'Health behaviors and psychosocial adjustment of migrant adolescents in Switzerland', Schweiz, *Medizinische Wochenschrift*, 127: 1419–29.

Fontana, E. and Beran, M. (1995) 'Sexuality and exclusion', *Revue Medical de la Suisse Romande*, 115: 495–7.

Ford, S. and Kittisuksathit, S. (1996) 'Sexual hazards for migrant workers', *World Heath Forum*, 17: 283–5.

Gfroerer, J. and Tan, L. (2003) 'Substance use among foreign-born youths in the United States: does the length of residence matter?' *American Journal of Public Health*, 93: 1892–6.

Haour-Knipe, M. (2001) *Moving Families: Expatriation, Stress and Coping*, London: Routledge.

Harrell-Bond, B. (2000) 'Are refugee camps good for children', *Journal of Humanitarian Assistance*. Working Paper No. 29. Online. Available HTTP: <http://www.jha.ac/articles/u029.htm> (accessed 12 January 2005).

Hernandez, D. and Charney, E. (eds) (1998) *From Generation to Generation: The Health and Well-being of Children in Immigrant Families*, Washington, DC: National Academy Press.

Hong Kong Special Administrative Region (2000) *Report on the Hong Kong Special Administrative Region Under the Convention Against Torture and Other Cruel, Inhuman or Degrading Treatment or Punishment: Updating Report*. Online. Available HTTP: <http://www.hab.gov.hk/en/policy_responsibilities/the_rights_of_the_individuals/cat.htm> (accessed 20 October 2004).

Human Rights Watch (2002) *Nowhere to Turn: State Abuses of Unaccompanied Migrant Children by Spain and Morocco*, Report, vol. 14(4D). Online. Available HTTP: <http://www.hrw.org/reports/2002/spain-morocco/> (accessed 20 January 2005).

International Labour Organization (ILO) (2004) *Towards a Fair Deal for Migrant Workers in a Global Economy*, Report VI, International Labour Conference 92nd Session, Geneva: ILO. Online. Available HTTP: <http://www.ilo.org/public/english/standards/relm/ilc/ilc92/pdf/rep-vi.pdf> (accessed 21 October 2004).

International Organization for Migration (2001) *Trafficking in Unaccompanied Minors for Sexual Exploitation in the European Union*, May, Brussels: IOM.

International Organization for Migration (2003) *World Migration 2003: Managing Migration Challenges and Responses for People on the Move*, Geneva: IOM.

Johnson, T. (1996) 'Alcohol and drug use among displaced persons: an overview', *Substance Use and Misuse* 31: 1853–89.

Johnson, T., VanGeest, J. and Cho, Y. (2002) 'Migration and substance use: evidence from the U.S. national health interview survey', *Substance Use and Misuse* 37: 941–72.

McKay, L., Macintyre, S. and Ellaway, A. (2003) *Migration and Health: A Review of the International Literature*. Occasional Paper No. 12, MRC, Medical Research Council's Medical Sociology Unit – Public Health Research Unit, University of Glasgow, Glasgow, Scotland. Available HTTP: <http://www.msoc-mrc.gla.ac.uk/ Publications/pub/PDFs/Occasional-Papers/OP012.pdf> (accessed 13 February 2005).

Martens, J., Pieczkowski, M. and van Vuuren-Smyth, B. (2003) *Seduction, Sale and Slavery: Trafficking in Women and Children for Sexual Exploitation in Southern Africa*. Pretoria: IOM. Online. Available HTTP: <http://www.iom.org.za/Reports/TraffickingReport3rdEd.pdf>

Martin, S.F. (2004) *Women and Migration*, Paper prepared for the United Nations

Division for the Advancement of Women Consultative Meeting on 'Migration and Mobility and how this Movement affects Women', CM/MMW/2003/WP, New York: United Nations.

Nantulya, V.M. *et al.* (2001) 'Tanzania: Gaining Insights into Adolescent Lives and Livelihoods.' Online. Available HTTP: <http://www.rockfound.org/Documents/424/chapter12.doc> (accessed 20 January 2005).

Nduna, S. and Goodyear, L. (1997) 'Pain too Deep for Tears: Assessing the Prevalence of Sexual and Gender Violence Among Burundian Refugees in Tanzania.' International Rescue Committee. Online. Available HTTP: <http://intranet.theirc.org/docs/sgbv_1.pdf> (accessed 14 February 2005).

Nemayechi, G. and Taveaux, T. (1997) *Harm Reduction Program for Vietnamese Drug Users in Pillar Point Refugee Camps.* Unpublished report prepared for Médecins Sans Frontières, Hong Kong.

Physicians for Human Rights (2004) 'Migration, Trafficking and the Exploitation of Women in Thailand.' Boston, MA: Physicians for Human Rights. Online. Available HTTP: <http://www.phrusa.org/campaigns/aids/pdf/nostatus.pdf>

Pick, W. and Cooper, D. (1997) 'Urbanisation and women's health in South Africa', *African Journal of Reproductive Health*, 1: 45–55.

Shaw, C. and Aggleton, P. (2002) *Preventing HIV/AIDS and Promoting Sexual Health Among Especially Vulnerable Young People*, Southampton: University of Southampton, Safe Passages to Adulthood Programme.

Shtarkshall, R. and Soskolne, V. (2000) *Migrant Populations and HIV/AIDS. The Development and Implementation of Programmes: Theory, Methodology and Practice*, Jerusalem: UNESCO/UNAIDS.

Turner, S. (1999) 'Angry young men in camps: gender, age and class relations among Burundian refugees in Tanzania', *Journal of Humanitarian Assistance*, Working Paper No. 9. Online. Available HTTP: <http://www.unhcr.ch/cgi-bin/texis/vtx/home/+NwwBmemmJ69wwwwowwwwwwwhFqo20I0E2gltFqoGn5nwGqrAFqo20I0E2glcFqtR1GDnGDzmxwwwwwww/opendoc.pdf> (accessed 14 February 2005).

United Nations Children's Fund (2001) *UNICEF Warns: Demand for Child Sex is Linked to Spread of HIV/AIDS*, Press Release CF/DOC/PR/2001-93, Geneva: UNICEF.

United Nations Development Programme (UNDP) (2003) *From Challenges to Opportunities: Responses to Trafficking and HIV/AIDS in South Asia.* New Delhi, UNDP Regional HIV and Development Programme, South and North East Asia. Online. Available HTTP: <http://www.youandaids.org/UNDP_REACH_publications/From%20Challenges%20to%20Opportunities/index.asp> (accessed 12 February 2005).

United Nations High Commission for Refugees (UNHCR) (2004) *2003 Global Refugee Trends*, Geneva: Population Data Unit, UNHCR.

United Nations Office for the Coordination of Humanitarian Affairs (2004) 'Afghanistan: Women and Addiction.' Online. Available HTTP: <http://216.239.59.104/search?q=cache:wa1NX4wP6awJ:www.plusnews.org/webspecials/opium/addfem.asp+Afghanistan+AND+women+AND+refugee+AND+heroinandhl=fr> (accessed 4 February 2004).

Vega, W.A., Zimmerman, R., Warheit, G. and Gil, A. (2003) 'Acculturation, stress and Latino adolescent drug use.' In *Socioeconomic Conditions, Stress and Mental*

Disorders: Toward a new Synthesis of Research and Public Policy, Collection of Working Papers, Chapter 9. Online. Available HTTP: <http://www.mhsip.org/nimhdoc/socioeconmh_home2.htm> (accessed 15 January 2004).

Verdurmen, J.E., Smit, F., Toet, J., *Van* Driel, H.F. and van Ameijden, E.J.C. (2004) 'Under-utilisation of addiction treatment services by heroin users from ethnic minorities: results from a cohort study over four years', *Addiction Research and Theory*, 12(3): 285.

Wijngaart, G.F. van de (1997) 'Drug problems among immigrants and refugees in the Netherlands and the Dutch health care and treatment system', *Substance Use and Misuse*, 32 (7 and 8): 909–38.

Willis, B.M. and Levy, B.S. (eds) (2002) 'Childhood prostitution: global health burden, research needs, and interventions', *The Lancet*, 339: 1417–22.

Women's Commission for Refugee Women and Children (2004) *Youth Speak Out: New Voices on the Protection and Participation of Young People Affected by Armed Conflict*. Online. Available HTTP: <http://www.womenscommission.org/pdf/cap_ysofinal_rev.pdf> (Accessed 6 February 2005).

Zafar, T., Brahmbhatt, H., Imam, G., Hassan, S. and Strathdee, S. (2003) 'HIV knowledge and risk behaviours among Pakistani and Afghani drug users in Quetta, Pakistan', *Journal of Acquired Immune Deficiency Syndromes*, April, 32(4): 394–8.

Zimmerman, C., Yun, K., Shvab, I., Watts, C., Trappolin, L., Treppete, M., Bimbi, F., Adams, B., Jiraporn, S., Beci, L., Albrecht, M., Bindel, J. and Regan, L. (2003) *The Health Risks and Consequences of Trafficking in Women and Adolescents: Findings from a European Study*. London: London School of Hygiene and Tropical Medicine. Available HTTP: <http://www.lshtm.ac.uk/hpu/docs/traffickingfinal.pdf> (accessed 12 February 2005).

Chapter 11

Young people, the military, sex and drugs

Martin Foreman

Over 20 million people serve in the armed forces across the world, the vast majority of them men. In times of widespread conflict, the total number under arms can rise considerably: in 1985 as many as 28 million people were estimated to be on active service (Project Ploughshares 2003). It is uncertain how many soldiers[1] are under 25 years old, although the figure is likely to be around 50 per cent. Each year over a million young people enter or leave military service.

The world's armed forces share many similarities – in addition to being relatively young in age and overwhelmingly male, they are highly hierarchical and highly mobile. There are also considerable differences determined by rates of pay, the conditions in which soldiers live and work, and whether the military comprises only of volunteers or has a high proportion of conscripts. All these factors influence soldiers' attitudes and experiences, both in and out of uniform.

While there are many anecdotal reports of soldiers' sexual behaviour and consumption of drugs and alcohol, statistics are less accessible. Some countries, particularly in Africa, do not release any such information and, where studies are published, different methodologies can make accurate comparison between countries difficult. Information from several parts of the world is missing from this analysis. Furthermore, where statistics are available, the behaviour of younger soldiers (under 25 years old) is seldom disaggregated from that of older servicemen and women.[2] Wherever possible, therefore, examples are taken from armies with a large conscript base, since most conscripted soldiers are under 25.

---

1 For the sake of brevity, in this chapter unless otherwise stated, references to soldiers include men and women serving in any of the armed forces, such as the navy and air force.

2 Exceptions include the US military, which analyses and provides some age-specific information, and the Royal Thai Army, which carries out yearly sample surveys of the sexual behaviour and alcohol consumption of serving conscripts, almost all of whom are between 21 and 25.

Despite the scarcity of statistics, however, there is enough information to draw four broad conclusions: military life can have a significant impact on young people's social, psychological and sexual development; in many, if not most, military forces young people are more sexually active than civilians of the same age; a significant proportion of young soldiers drink heavily; and, with some exceptions, illicit drug use is probably not widespread among young soldiers.

Age and background

Soldiers usually enlist in their late teens or early twenties. Most conscripts, who are almost always male, finish their military service by their twenty-fifth birthday, while volunteers – also known as career soldiers – may stay until their forties or fifties. This means that all-volunteer armies tend to have a higher age profile than those with conscripts. Officers, who receive significantly longer and more in-depth training than the ranks, are likely to enter at a slightly later age, depending on the entry requirements of the particular force they are joining, and to remain in active service longer.

The age of new recruits has risen steadily in recent years. The international Optional Protocol to the Convention on the Rights of the Child outlaws the direct involvement of children under 18 in hostilities and bars compulsory recruitment below that age. However, in warfare, both insurgent and government forces may recruit younger teenagers and even children. Some 300,000 child soldiers are currently estimated to be involved in armed conflict in combat or non-combat roles, including as sex partners; and many are recruited by force.

Whether conscripts or volunteers, soldiers in the ranks tend to come from a poorer background and to be less educated than the general population. This may also mean that members of a country's ethnic minorities may be over-represented, if their standard of living is lower than that of the majority ethnic group. For example, 18–28 per cent of the different branches of the US military are black, compared to 12 per cent in the general population.

A man's life

Women represent a minority in the global armed forces. Depending on definition (administrative positions may be considered members of the military), the ratio of women soldiers ranges from under one in a hundred, as in Cambodia, through 14 per cent, as in the USA, to one in three in the Eritrean army during its liberation war in the early 1990s. In only about a dozen countries do the armed forces grant women full combat status. Women tend to be found in higher numbers and are more likely to serve on the frontlines in insurgent forces, as in El Salvador and Nicaragua in the 1980s and Eritrea in the 1990s.

Despite the presence of women, the predominant culture in the world's armed forces is that to be a soldier is to be a man. Although concepts of masculinity vary between and within cultures, they almost always include a common core of physical prowess and the ability to overcome one's opponent, attributes which are prized in the armed forces.

The link between masculinity and sexual activity is also strong and consistently present in soldiers' daily banter. One US military chant goes 'This is my rifle, this is my gun. My rifle's for killing, my gun is for fun.' The masculine ethos means that women in the armed forces may have to exert considerable effort to prove themselves as good as men physically and emotionally, on the training ground and in battle.

Living conditions

The physical and psychological conditions in which soldiers live vary widely. In wealthier countries, barracks may offer comparative comfort, while in the poorest countries they are often overcrowded, with sleeping, washing and other facilities stretched to the point of squalor. Living conditions for Russian conscripts, who comprise upwards of 1 million men, are widely reported to be among the worst in the world, with such basic amenities as an adequate diet and washing facilities lacking. Common rooms may be absent, poorly maintained or their use restricted to officers or other privileged soldiers. 'Soldiers have nothing here, no activity, nothing. There's no exercise room; one TV set, that's all', said one Slovak conscript (Bianchi 2000: 118). A key element of most soldiers' lives is lack of privacy, which in some cases extends to the most basic functions of hygiene and excretion.

Recognising that barracks life can lead to tedium and tension, most military authorities provide distractions and entertainment such as sports and films, although the budget for such facilities may be limited. Some militaries, such as the Indian army, encourage activities such as mountaineering, white water rafting, skiing or parachuting, which can also find operational use. Where there are few distractions, soldiers tend to devise other ways of spending their time, such as games with weapons. Such activities are a means of reasserting individual autonomy and identity in a disempowering environment.

Soldiers are frequently stationed away from their base, on exercise, on peacekeeping missions or during conflict. A posting with few responsibilities but a range of facilities may relieve tensions, while posting to a conflict zone or a poorly populated area with few diversions may compound them.

Loving or loathing it

Young people enter the armed forces at a formative stage in their lives. For many, this may be the first time that they are away for an extended period

from their families and communities. They have to live in new social structures – not only the formal hierarchy of the military, but twenty-four hours
a day, seven days a week among their peers. Their attitudes and opinions
about the world around them and their place in it are still being formed, and
from an environment where many voices may be heard – their parents, their
friends, schoolteachers, the media etc. – they move to an environment where
the strongest voice is of the peer group in which they live.

Volunteers may not know what to expect, but they enter this world
willingly and are usually more able to adapt. They expect to benefit from
military service, through their own efforts and the career opportunities
offered. In addition to the benefit of increased self-esteem, long-term soldiers
can expect to gather a range of skills that can eventually be taken into civilian
life, to see their income improve, and to move into married quarters that offer
greater privacy and comfort.

Many conscripts, however, often view military service as an unwelcome
interruption, at best depriving them of career and/or education opportunities
and restricting their social and sexual lives, and at worst imposing months
or years of physical discomfort, fear and constant humiliation. On the other
hand, some conscripts, particularly those from disadvantaged backgrounds,
may welcome military service. In Honduras in the 1980s, when forced
conscription of young men was common, life in the armed forces was harsh
and sometimes brutal. Nevertheless, for many rural youths it was their first
opportunity to receive new clothes, a balanced diet, medical treatment and
the opportunity to learn to read (Library of Congress 1995). For these and
other young men with limited experience and searching for an identity for
themselves, military life can offer both security and a means of developing
that identity.

The very different psychological and physical circumstances in which
soldiers find themselves mean that the range of emotions they experience
varies widely. Activities designed to build communal spirit and mutual
support may succeed or may alienate. Warfare can exhilarate or terrify.
Individual soldiers may experience comradeship, excitement, arrogance
and a sense of invulnerability or low self-esteem, fear, boredom and extreme
loneliness. While older, career soldiers are more likely to have the experience
to deal with such emotions, younger soldiers often have few resources with
which to respond, particularly to the negative aspects of military life.

Alcohol and tobacco

Both legal and illegal recreational drugs enhance experience and improve
mood. They are therefore attractive to young soldiers seeking a means of
reducing the stresses of military life. In the armed forces worldwide, alcohol
and tobacco are the most commonly consumed substances.

Except in those few countries where the sale and consumption of alcohol is illegal in all circumstances, the availability of alcohol in the military varies. On military bases it may be forbidden, or usually confined to specific sites or allowed to officers but not the ranks. Despite these restrictions, however, alcohol is usually easily accessed. It may be sold on base, often at a subsidised price, or available in nearby shops and bars. And when soldiers drink, reasons can be easily found to consume large quantities: to celebrate a birthday, to commemorate a companion, or simply because they are on leave.

Young soldiers tend to be particularly heavy drinkers. In the United States in 1998, 15 per cent of all soldiers reported heavy alcohol drinking (defined as five or more drinks in one day at least 12 times during the past 12 months). Among 18–25 year olds, the figure was 27 per cent, compared with 15 per cent of civilians in the same age group (SAMHSA 2002). In Slovakia, where conscripts comprise slightly more than half the armed forces,

> alcohol consumption, although officially forbidden in the barracks, is in practice generally accepted. If this prohibition is broken, it is punished as only a minor disciplinary offence. A soldier returning to the barracks under the influence of alcohol is isolated only if his behaviour is openly violent.
>
> (Bianchi and Popper 2000: 759)

Forty-two per cent of Slovak soldiers say they drink alcohol 'socially' at least once a week; and 11 per cent drink 'heavily' (with loss of self-control) during the same period (Bianchi and Popper 2000: 760).

Sex and alcohol are closely linked. When sex is desired but not available, alcohol can relieve the desire; and when sex is available, alcohol can fuel it. In the early 1990s, many Thai military conscripts (almost all of whom are 21–23 years old) reported drinking for fun, to reduce inhibitions both with women and with their fellow soldiers, and to increase sexual pleasure. Alcohol was strongly associated with visits to sex workers, which played a strong role in social bonding both outside and within the army (MacQueen *et al.* 1996). Although visits to sex work establishments have fallen across Thailand in the last ten years, drinking persists in alternative venues, such as karaoke bars, where sex is still available.

Tobacco fulfils a similar role to alcohol in many armed forces. Smoking not only brings desired physical sensations but fills in free time and is a symbol of comradeship. Cigarettes may be used by officers as a means of encouraging soldiers to relax, and soldiers who do not smoke may be excluded from some social groups. Where statistics are available, the extent of tobacco consumption in the military appears to reflect that in the civilian population. In the USA in 1998, 30 per cent of all soldiers admitted smoking cigarettes, compared to the civilian rate of 33 per cent (SAMHSA 2002).

Illicit drugs

Statistics are not widely available, but where they do exist, they suggest that illicit recreational drug use may be lower in the military than in the civilian population. This may be because prohibition is strongly enforced, because the price of drugs is beyond soldiers' means, or because a significant proportion of soldiers subscribe to the military ethos of hostility towards drug use. The drugs that are consumed tend to reflect local availability. They may include both internationally used substances such as marijuana/cannabis, cocaine, ecstasy and heroin and variations manufactured or processed according to local custom.

The US military has significantly reduced the extent of soldiers' drug use through education campaigns and strict enforcement of regulations through such methods as random urine tests and the deployment of sniffer dogs. Between 1980 and 1998, use of any illicit drug in the US armed forces fell from 27.6 per cent to 2.7 per cent, compared with a fall in the general population from 14 per cent in 1979 to 7 per cent in 2001. Among 18–25 year olds in the general population, the reported use of marijuana fell from 36 per cent to 16 per cent and of cocaine (including crack) from 10 per cent to 2 per cent in the same period (ONDCP 2002).

Similar measures are undertaken by the armed forces of other countries, while in countries where such widespread methods are not used to contain illicit drug use, military authorities may still consider it a serious problem despite evidence to the contrary. In Slovakia, the country's armed forces – more than half of whom are conscripts – automatically discharge any soldier found in possession or under the influence of an illegal substance, yet only 22 soldiers were treated for substance abuse in 1998, while, as pointed out above, excessive alcohol consumption was considerably more common (Bianchi and Popper 2000).

While use of illicit drugs appears uncommon among most young soldiers, the practice may be widespread in a few countries. Reports from Russia suggest that conscripts in the north Caucasus, where the army is active against insurgent forces, regularly use drugs to suppress stress and depression. And in 2002 Vasily Harchenko, an AIDS expert in the country's Ministry of Defence, claimed that at least 20 per cent of Russian soldiers diagnosed with HIV had taken drugs during their service (Rozovskaya 2002).

Legally supplied

In certain circumstances, some drugs may be tolerated or even made available by the military authorities to enhance fighting capacity. Since at least the Vietnam War, the US air force has made amphetamines (commonly known as speed) available to its crews to allow them to fly long hours, as well as sedatives to enable them to sleep once the amphetamine-enhanced mission is complete.

Despite occasional inappropriate consequences, including allegations that four Canadian soldiers died in Afghanistan as a result of the actions of a US pilot who had taken amphetamines and the use of officially prescribed drugs in cases where soldiers murdered their wives, the US continues to undertake research into chemical enhancement of soldiers' ability to perform in battle (Knickerbocker 2002).

Some insurgent forces supply drugs that are generally considered illicit. Since the early 1990s, *qat* (a plant bark chewed as a stimulant, also known as *miraa*) has been regularly flown in from Kenya to encourage the soldiers of different militia in Somalia to fight.

Sex

Sex is a preoccupation of many young male soldiers. In some countries, army life increases opportunities for sex, while in others it appears to reduce it. Access to sex depends not only on free time but often also on financial status – soldiers with money to spend appear more likely to have sexual partners than those who earn relatively little. Access to sex may also be affected by military policy. In the past, many armed forces recruited women, voluntarily or otherwise, to provide soldiers with sexual services; others tolerated the presence of brothels and camp-followers. Some insurgent forces, most notoriously the Lord's Revolutionary Army in northern Uganda, still kidnap women and children for this purpose.

Today, however, national armies are more likely to restrict access to sex on grounds of discipline, to reduce conflict with locals and/or to reduce the risks of contracting sexually transmitted infections. Soldiers' free time and leave may therefore be limited, and soldiers may be prohibited from visiting sex workers or areas where sex workers operate. In some cases, as in the Indian Army, all casual sex is prohibited, although no restrictions apply on home leave.

Long-term relationships may also be discouraged. In Zambia, soldiers are prevented from marrying for the first two years of service, after which the consent of a superior officer is required. The delay is necessary, according to Colonel Joyce Puta, formerly of the Zambian Defence Forces, partly so that younger soldiers can mature, and partly because they are likely to be sent on long tours of duty that would separate them from their spouses.

Restrictive measures are not universal and may not always be effective. In many countries, particularly in the developing world, military bases attract a large civilian presence, including places of entertainment where sex workers can be found.

Certain situations increase the likelihood of young soldiers having sex; for Slovakian conscripts – and no doubt young soldiers from many other countries – these include the first home leave ('sexual intercourse at all costs'), the second half of military service when visits to nightclubs and alcohol consumption are more common, being encouraged by fellow soldiers to lose one's virginity, and isolated workplaces with little supervision (Bianchi 2000). Additional factors identified in Ghana include: young people's tendency to perceive themselves as invulnerable, extra money paid during military operations and a host population dependent on the military for essentials such as food (Foreman 2002). The last two factors are particularly relevant in impoverished communities where male soldiers wield money and/or power; sex may be demanded from (or offered by) women in a variety of situations, from the short-term need for food or to pass through a checkpoint to the longer-term need to find shelter and security.

The association between the military and sex work persists in many countries – usually supplemented with alcohol, as in the example from Thailand above. In many parts of Africa, there are few places where only sex is sold, but many bars where barmaids make much of their income from selling sex. Sex may also be available on military bases from women providing services such as cooking or laundry, or from the wives of other soldiers. The major problem on base is privacy; to overcome this, there may be a tradition of soldiers vacating a dormitory to allow one to have sex with a regular partner, or casual partners may be shared.

Given these factors, it is not surprising that the statistics available show a correlation between men's military service and their access to sex. While studies in the general population in many countries show that up to one in three men in their late teens and early twenties has more than one sexual partner a year; the figure appears consistently higher for soldiers in many countries, including Belgium (Wouters 1995), France (Whiteside 1996), the Netherlands (Groennings 1997) and the United Kingdom (Whiteside 1996).

Where young soldiers' pay is lower than average, as in conscription-based armies in Eastern Europe and Latin America, opportunities for sex appear to diminish. Conscripts in Slovakia, who earn US$18 a month, compared to an average of $700 before enlisting (late 1990s figures), report less sex than in civilian life (Bianchi 2000) and complain that a military uniform – a sign of prestige in many countries – is a barrier to meeting women. Russian conscripts are even more poorly paid, with monthly pay in 2002 between 60 and 100 roubles (US$2–3).

Yet even in lower income countries the reality may be different. Research in Slovakia identified three groups of women who specifically seek sex with young soldiers: girls aged 12 to 16, particularly in rural areas; divorced or sexually unsatisfied women over 30; and ethnic minority Roma, who have very low socio-economic status (Bianchi 2000).

Women soldiers

Little statistical information is available about the sex lives of young women soldiers. Anecdotal evidence suggests that young women soldiers are not as active in seeking sexual intercourse as their male colleagues. However, some are sexually active. Unofficial reports from the US army suggested relatively high rates of pregnancy during the first (1990–1991) Gulf War.

While young women's sexual partners are likely to be civilians, sex between male and female soldiers does occur. During the Eritrean war of liberation in the 1990s, when a third of the armed forces were women serving in the same, often extremely hazardous, conditions as men, consensual sexual relations between the sexes were relatively common. In Israel, which conscripts both men and women at the age of 18, and the USA, which has an all-volunteer force, anecdotal reports of sex between male and female soldiers are not unknown.

There are widespread reports of sexual harassment (which does not include physical abuse) and rape of women soldiers by other soldiers in the US military – with one study suggesting that up to one in four had been subject to sexual assault (Murdoch and Nichol 1995: 414). Lower rates have been reported by US servicewomen returning from service in Iraq in 2003–2004 (Moffeit and Herdy 2004). Similar anecdotal reports come from other countries. And girl soldiers (under 18 years old) in both government and insurgent armed forces are frequently subject to sexual exploitation by colleagues and commanders. Twenty-eight per cent 'provide' sexual services, according to one survey (Alfredson n.d.; McKay and Mazurana n.d.).

Between men

While strong emotional bonds among soldiers boost morale, in most countries male soldiers who are known to have sex with men are almost always punished and often discharged. In a few countries, such as Australia and the Netherlands, men who identify as gay – preferring emotional and sexual relationships with other men – are welcomed into the armed forces. Irrespective of policy, however, sex between men does occur – either between two soldiers or between a soldier and a civilian.

Anecdotal evidence includes a group of Peruvian soldiers recalling several cases of officers having sex with recruits, and a Thai air force trainee pilot reporting several incidents of sexual abuse of young colleagues known to be or suspected of being gay. In Zambia, however, one interview group claimed there is no sex between male soldiers, partly because of strong taboos, and partly because two men would never have the opportunity to be alone together (Foreman 2002).

Sexual abuse by other male soldiers does occur. One report from the USA suggests that at least 22,000 men were subject to some form of sexual abuse in the last forty years. 'Sexual assaults on military men is much more prevalent than people imagine,' says a veterans' counsellor. 'In basic training, it's easy to exert one's power over a young recruit.' Investigations into abuse of male soldiers have found widespread denial of the problem (Snel 2003).

Meanwhile, the abuse of boy soldiers (under 18), has also been reported although not widely investigated (Alfredson n.d.).

Outside the barracks, sex with men may provide soldiers with extra income. There are many reports of conscripted soldiers selling sex in the United Kingdom and USA in the first half of the twentieth century. Of today's conscripts, Chilean researcher and former director of Corporación Chilena de Prevención del SIDA, Tim Frasca, writes 'low pay makes it difficult for soldiers to visit women sex workers, so they sometimes accept alternatives among local men, which may not only be free but include drinks, food, lodging and even a relationship. Most return to heterosexual lives when they leave the army.' Similar experiences are reported from Peru, while in Slovakia conscripts report that half a month's pay or more can be made from one encounter with a client.

In time of war

During wartime, attitudes towards death and survival and perceptions of risk change. Among both civilians and soldiers casual sex is encouraged by the attitude that 'I might die tomorrow, so I should live today.' Overall, rates of consensual sex and rape rise – one study reports systematic rape of women and children by soldiers in over 20 countries across the world in the last 30 years (Seagar 1997).

Opportunities for sex in wartime depend on such factors as the nature of the conflict and the extent of discipline in the armed forces. Warfare that uses technologically advanced weaponry allows few opportunities for soldiers and civilians to meet. Fighting that depends mostly on infantry provides different scenarios, including periods of intense conflict where there are no opportunities or desire for sex, lulls which allow opportunities for sex with civilians or other soldiers, and periods of high tension where women and girls, and sometimes men and boys, are raped. However, while there are many anecdotal stories about sex in times of war, there appears to be no conclusive evidence as to the particular impact of warfare on the sexual or drug-taking activity of young soldiers.

Implications

While military life can be beneficial for some young people, it can also have negative consequences. These may be as severe as serious injury or death – in combat, in accidents or the result of suicide by individuals unable to adapt to military life. Unprotected sexual intercourse can lead to high rates of sexually transmitted infections (STIs). Consumption of alcohol may underlie many such incidents.

Soldiers' relative freedom of movement and association with civilian populations during times of peace and war has placed them at the centre of

STI epidemics for at least the last five hundred years, with infection rates usually higher in units far from home. In the 1830s, at least one in three British soldiers stationed in India was hospitalised for an STI, compared to one in 30 Indian soldiers, a pattern that continued for over half a century. During the 1960s, rates of infection among US soldiers in Vietnam – many of whom were conscripts – were nine times higher than among those based at home; during the same period in Thailand, where many US soldiers spent their leave, almost one in two contracted an STI and rates were fifteen times higher than in the USA (World Bank 1999).

Even domestic rates tend to be higher than in the civilian population. In the USA in 1998, syphilis incidence was two to three times higher in the marines, army and navy than in the general public; only the air force rate was lower (McGinn *et al.* 2001). In 1996, the Chlamydia rate among women soldiers in the USA was three to six times that of the general population (Moffeit and Herdy 2004).

HIV/AIDS

In some parts of the world, particularly sub-Saharan Africa, HIV rates are often higher in the armed forces than in the general population. Late 1990s estimates include 40–60 per cent of Angolan soldiers being HIV-positive (compared with 3 per cent of the adult population), 10–25 per cent in Congo (Brazzaville) (cf. 6 per cent), 5 per cent in Eritrea (cf. 2 per cent) (UNAIDS 2003), 15–30 per cent in Tanzania (cf. 9 per cent) and 50 per cent in Zimbabwe (cf. 25 per cent) (Hsu 2001). In Cambodia in 1999, 12–17 per cent of the armed forces were estimated to be HIV-positive, compared with 4 per cent of the general population (Cochrane 1999). Given the low incidence of injecting drug use in the armed forces, such rates are almost always the result of sexual activity, although transfusion of contaminated blood and shared skin-piercing instruments, such as razors and tattoo needles, may also be implicated.

The armed forces may also be implicated in the spread of HIV in the civilian population. Where soldiers have a limited choice of partners, men from the same company or ship are likely to have sex with the same women over a period of time; when that company is replaced, the new soldiers have intercourse with the same women. Even if only a small number of soldiers or their partners have a disease at the beginning of the process, frequent sex without a condom will soon cause the infection to spread. In northern Namibia, infection rates significantly higher than the national average were confirmed in communities close to military bases in the 1990s (Webb 1997: 104–6). And in a 1999 study in northern Uganda, more than one in three of a group of widows living with HIV/AIDS had a soldier as their last sexual partner (Abwola and Dolan 1999).

However, many armed forces now show lower rates of HIV infection than in the general population. This frequently reflects a policy of screening potential recruits and/or serving members, excluding, downgrading or dismissing those found to be HIV-positive and/or intensive education campaigns, often carried out in partnership with international organisations. As a result of such campaigns, in Morocco where conscripts make up half the armed forces, estimated HIV infection rates were three in 10,000 in the general adult population in 1999, compared with two in 100,000 in the army; the incidence of other STIs in the armed forces fell from over 5,000 cases a year in 1987 to 3,000 by 1996 (Nejmi *et al.* 2000). In Ethiopia, the HIV infection rate of 5 per cent in the armed forces is 2 per cent lower than in the general population (Tidwell 2002). And in Thailand, another conscript-based military, where the government has encouraged sex workers and clients to use condoms consistently, HIV infection among soldiers dropped from 12 per cent in 1993 to under 3 per cent in 1998. Soldiers' visits to sex workers dropped from 80 to 38 per cent in the same period (Johns Hopkins University 2002).

In other words, soldiers' sexual behaviour appears to be changing. Whether that change differs by age is unclear, but it is likely that in many countries young soldiers are currently less sexually active than their predecessors. Furthermore, whether that change is long term is also uncertain. Each year, a new batch of young men and women enters the armed forces, bringing with them their own ideas as to appropriate sexual behaviour – ideas that continue to change under the influence of the mass media, including ever-increasing access to the internet and sexually explicit materials.

Conclusions

Young people form the backbone of the armed forces in every country of the world. Even in volunteer militaries, men and women under 25 years old are likely to comprise almost half the fighting force. Young people in the military tend to come from relatively deprived backgrounds, both in terms of wealth and education. Their attitudes towards sex and recreational drugs are frequently ones of curiosity and experimentation. Their sexual and drug-taking behaviour is strongly influenced by both the military hierarchy and peer pressure, sometimes working in harmony (perceptions of masculinity) and sometimes in opposition (the acceptability of illicit drugs).

While there is little published information on young women in the military, there is enough evidence to show that young men tend to be more sexually active than their civilian peers, and to drink more alcohol – which often fuels their sexual activity. There is also a strong link in many countries between the military and sex work, with some soldiers regularly buying sex and others selling it.

Sex in itself is not harmful, nor is sex work, but too often the sexual situations in which soldiers find themselves are not ideal and not conducive to protecting themselves or their partners from disease. Similarly, moderate alcohol use can have benefits, but excess can be both physically and mentally harmful. Meanwhile, recreational drug use tends to be lower, except in insurgent forces and militaries where pay is low, boredom widespread, discipline erratic and drugs relatively accessible.

Some young people are well suited to military life and benefit from it; others are physically or mentally scarred. While conscription remains a fact of life in many countries, there is slow movement in some, for example Russia, to move to an all-volunteer army. Such a step will be beneficial to the thousands of young people who consider that the time spent in the armed forces is time stolen from their lives.

But whatever the basis under which they serve, young people in many militaries lack the opportunities to develop appropriate and healthy attitudes and behaviour towards sex, alcohol and recreational drugs. Steps that have been taken in some armed forces to encourage peer-led education on HIV and STIs need to be expanded and in some cases the attitudes of the military hierarchy towards sex, alcohol and drugs need to be re-examined.

References

Abwola, S. and Dolan, C. (1999) 'HIV and Conflict in Gulu District: Findings from an ACORD Study.' Paper presented at an international conference on 'Peace research and reconciliation agenda', Gulu, Uganda, 27–29 September.

Alfredson, L. (n.d.) *Sexual Exploitation of Child Soldiers: An Exploration and Analysis of Global Dimensions and Trends*, Coalition to Stop the Use of Child Soldiers. Online. Available HTTP: <http://www.child-soldiers.org/cs/childsoldiers. nsf/0/36fdc21ed10c9b1380256b27003bdaa1?OpenDocument>

Bianchi, G. (2000) *A Rapid Situation Assessment of Substance Use and Sexual Risk Behaviour in Slovakia*, Bratislava: Department of Social and Biological Communication, Slovak Academy of Sciences.

Bianchi, G. and Popper, M. (2000) 'Interaction of substance use and risks to sexual health in the Slovak Army: general, socio-cultural, and individual behaviour patterns', *AIDS Care*, 12: 757–66.

Cochrane, J. (1999) 'Troops face unseen enemy as HIV sweeps through ranks', *South China Morning Post*, 31 March and SEA-AIDS listserv [2162] 21 September 1999.

Foreman, M. (2002) *Combat AIDS: HIV and the World's Armed Forces*, London: Healthlink Worldwide. Online. Available HTTP: <http://www.healthlink.org.uk/ COMBAT%20AIDS%20PDF.pdf>

Groennings, S. (ed.) (1997) *HIV/AIDS Strategy in Latin America and Africa: Military and Civil–Military Policies and Issues*, Hanover, New Hampshire: USA Civil–Military Alliance to Combat HIV and AIDS.

Hsu, L.-N. (2001) *HIV Subverts National Security*, Bangkok: UNDP, South East Asia HIV and Development Project.

Johns Hopkins University (2002) *The Gazette Online*, Vol. 21, No. 28. Online. Available HTTP: <www.jhu.edu/~gazette/2002/01apr02/01condom.html> (accessed 31 March 2004).

Knickerbocker, B. (2002) 'Military looks to drugs for battle readiness', *The Christian Science Monitor*, 9 August. Online. Available HTTP: <http://www.csmonitor.com/ 2002/0809/p01s04-usmi.html> (accessed 9 January 2004).

Library of Congress, Federal Research Division (1995) *Country Studies: Honduras*, Washington, DC. Online. Available HTTP: <http://lcweb2.loc.gov/frd/cs/hntoc. html>, subsection 'The Armed Forces: Recruitment and Training' or <http:// reference.allrefer.com/country-guide-study/honduras/honduras131.html> (accessed 31 March 2004).

McGinn, T., Purdin, S.J., Krause, S. and Jones, R.K. (2001) *Forced Migration and Transmission of HIV and Other Sexually Transmitted Infections: Policy and Programmatic Responses*, HIV InSite Knowledge Base Chapter. Online. Available HTTP: <http://hivinsite.ucsf.edu/InSite?page=kb-08-01-08> (accessed 13 October 2004).

McKay, S. and Mazurana, D. (n.d) *Girls in Militaries, Paramilitaries, and Armed Opposition Groups*, Canada: War Affected Children website. Online. Available HTTP: <http://www.waraffectedchildren.gc.ca/girls-en.asp> (accessed 13 October 2004).

MacQueen, K.M., Nopkesorn, T., Sweat, M.D., Sawaengdee, Y., Mastro, T.D. and Weniger, B.G. (1996) 'Alcohol consumption, brothel attendance and condom use: normative expectations among Thai military conscripts', *Medical Anthropology Quarterly*, 10: 402–23.

Moffeit, M. and Herdy, A. (2004) 'Returning female GIs report rapes, poor care', *Denver Post*, 25 January. Online. Available HTTP: <http://www.denverpost.com/ Stories/0,1413,36~6439~1913069,00.html> (accessed 10 April 2004).

Murdoch, M. and Nichol, K.L. (1995) 'Women veterans' experiences with domestic violence and with sexual harassment while in the military', *Archives of Family Medicine*, 4 (May): 411–18.

Nejmi, S., Sekkat, A., Oualine, M., Belekbir, M., Belafqih, L., Jirary, A., Ghidinelli, M.N., Monassif, M., Benghabrit, M. and Molato, A. (2000) 'Preventing STI HIV/AIDS through extensive IEC among the royal armed forces of the kingdom of Morroco', Abstracts of XIII International AIDS Conference, Durban. Online. Available HTTP: <http://www.iac2000.org/abdetail.asp?ID=TuPpD1183>

ONDCP (2002) *Fact Sheet: Drug Use Trends,* October. Drug Policy Information Clearinghouse, Executive Office of the President/Office of National Drug Control Policy, USA. Online. Available HTTP: <http://www.whitehousedrugpolicy.gov/ publications/factsht/druguse/drugusetrends.pdf> (accessed 9 January 2004).

Project Ploughshares (2003) *Swords and Ploughshares*, Waterloo, Canada. Online. Available HTTP: <http://www.ploughshares.ca/CONTENT/BUILD%20PEACE/ swordsandploughshares.pdf> (accessed 12 December 2003).

Rozovskaya, L. (2002) 'See a prostitute? Where would we find the money?', unpublished paper.

SAMHSA (2002) *National Survey on Drug Use and Health: National Findings Appendix E*, Rockville, USA: US Department of Health and Human Services. Online. Available HTTP: <http://www.oas.samhsa.gov/oas/nhsda/2k2nsduh/ Results/appE.htm> (accessed 31 March 2004).

Seagar, J. (1997) *The State of Women in the World Atlas*, New York: Penguin Books.

Snel, A. (2003) 'Male sex abuse revealed in ranks', *Florida Today*, 19 January 2003.

Tidwell, M. (2002) 'Ethiopia strives to control HIV', *Baltimore Sun*, 8 March.

Online. Available HTTP: <http://www.thebody.com/cdc/news_updates_archive/
mar8_02/ethiopia_aids.html> (accessed 13 October 2004).

UNAIDS (2003) *Fighting AIDS: HIV/AIDS Prevention and Care Among Armed
Forces and UN Peacekeepers: The Case of Eritrea*, Copenhagen: UNAIDS Series:
Engaging uniformed services in the fight against AIDS Case Study 1.

Webb, D. (1997) *HIV and AIDS in Africa*, Pluto Press, London.

Whiteside, A. (1996) 'HIV/AIDS in the armed forces', *Civil Military Alliance
Newsletter*, 2: 2.

World Bank (1999) *Policy Research Report: Confronting AIDS*, New York: Oxford
University Press.

Wouters, R. (1995) 'Belgian Military Medicine, AIDS: No Cure, but Care',
Civil–Military Alliance Newsletter, 1(2): 6.

Chapter 12

Young people in detention

Jan Copeland, John Howard and Anthony Arcuri

All over the world, young people find themselves detained in a controlled environment in a number of ways and under a variety of circumstances. More than 1 million children worldwide have been deprived of their liberty by law enforcement authorities and officials (UNICEF n.d.). Contexts in which young people may be detained include adult jails, juvenile detention centres, community group homes, re-education camps, labour camps, refugee camps, orphanages, and mandatory residential mental health or drug treatment programmes.

Despite the United Nations adoption of the Beijing Rules in 1985, outlining minimum standards for the administration of juvenile justice internationally, there is much to be concerned about with regard to the detention of young people.[1] It is widely understood that children and young people not infrequently experience violence at the hands of police and other law enforcement officials. Street children, in particular, may be especially vulnerable because they are poor, young, often unaware of their rights, and lack financial means and social support from an adult. Many thousands of children and young people are abandoned in orphanages and other non-penal institutions where they may be subject to abuse and neglect with no legal protection (Human Rights Watch 2001).

Young people in detention often suffer severe violations of their human rights. Detained children below the age of criminal responsibility may be kept with adult prisoners who may abuse them. A significant number of children in detention have not committed a criminal act but are deprived of their liberty as a result of 'status offences' such as vagrancy, begging or truancy. Young people may also be detained because they are accompanying a parent

---

1 The Beijing Rules refer to a comprehensive social policy that aims at promoting the welfare of young people to the greatest possible extent by minimising intervention by the juvenile justice system, promoting diversion from custody, and reducing the harm caused by any intervention (OHCHR 1985). They are supported by United Nations Rules for the Protection of Juveniles Deprived from their Liberty.

in detention or seeking asylum in another country, or in some instances simply because of their race, religion, nationality, ethnicity or political views (UNICEF n.d.).

In some countries, young people may be held in custody because they have possessed and/or used drugs. In some developing countries, children and young people make up a significant minority of those in often large, overcrowded, poorly staffed and poorly run detention facilities for the 'compulsory treatment' of drug users. Such placement increases their vulnerability and heightens the risk of various forms of abuse, substance use, unprotected sexual activity, blood-borne and other infections, and diminished health status.

Western models of juvenile justice

Juvenile courts first appeared in Western countries at the beginning of the twentieth century (Feld 2003). With the passage of time, their status jurisdiction has, however, expanded beyond the strictly criminal to embrace non-criminal behaviours such as smoking, sexual activity, truancy, 'immorality' and 'living an idle and dissolute life'. In the early days at least, such courts not infrequently imposed indeterminate and non-proportional sentences characterised as treatment and supervision rather than punishment. By the 1970s, however, conservatives and liberals attacked such rehabilitative ideals, replacing them with ideologies of crime prevention through incarceration and punishment (Beale 2003).

Macro-structural, economic and racial demographic changes occurring in US cities during the 1970s and 1980s, and the escalation in Black youth homicide rates during that period led to the 'get tough' juvenile justice policies that emerged in the 1990s (Beale 2003). One factor contributing to this change was the epidemic of crack cocaine use in the USA, which acted as a trigger to gun violence and youth homicides (Feld 2003). In the USA and some other Western countries, the media and conservative politicians alike have demonised young people to muster support for wars on drugs and crime.

While most other countries have not experienced crack cocaine or gun homicide epidemics, there has nonetheless been a rising incidence in juvenile crime among certain populations of young people, alongside an overrepresentation of particular minority populations in criminal justice statistics possibly due to differential law enforcement. In Australia, for example, indigenous youth currently have a juvenile detention rate 16 to 19 times higher than that of other young Australians (AIHW 2003: 352).

One of the most vulnerable groups in detention are girls, whose numbers have dramatically increased. Girls are now the fastest growing sector of the US juvenile justice system (ABA 2001) and in Canada (Reitsma-Street 1999). Girls entering the juvenile justice system are often subjected to one or more forms of emotional, physical or sexual abuse, with 40 per cent reporting having been raped, 62 per cent reporting drug use and 50 per cent parental drug use (Physicians for Human Rights n.d.). The long-term outcomes for arrested and incarcerated girls include a high risk of substance dependence, psychiatric problems, HIV infection, poor physical health, domestic and other forms of violence, delivering substance exposed babies, losing custody of their children, incarceration and increased mortality (Lederman *et al.* 2004).

Developing and transitional countries

Many poorly resourced countries operate informal and unregulated juvenile justice systems with significant military and paramilitary involvement. Issues of concern in these contexts include children being detained by police or other authorities without sufficient cause, for too long, without notification to their parents or guardians, or simply as a mechanism of intimidation (Human Rights Watch 2001).

Human Rights Watch has documented systemic failures to guarantee children legal representation and otherwise provide fair hearings in Brazil, Bulgaria, Guatemala, India, Jamaica, Pakistan, Russia and the United States (Human Rights Watch 2004). In Russia, for example, homeless young people have been apprehended and placed in collection/redistribution centres that were subsequently closed down because of concerns about human rights and illegal detention (Human Rights Watch 1998).

Violence in detention is also well documented among young people. This includes corporal punishment, torture, isolation, restraint, sexual assault, harassment and humiliation. In Kenya, for example, some young people in detention complained of excessive corporal punishment involving naked caning in public for homosexual acts, trying to escape, or smoking tobacco or cannabis (Human Rights Watch 2001).

A particular concern for young people in detention in developing and transitional countries is HIV infection, particularly through injecting drug use (Ball, Rana and Dehne 1998). A wide range of HIV prevention strategies have been implemented in developing countries and countries in transition. They include opioid substitution pharmacotherapy, needle and syringe exchange and distribution, condom and bleach distribution, outreach to injecting drug users (IDUs), peer education programmes, and social network interventions. However, in most settings these are not widely available to young people in detention, despite the increased risks if detained in custodial settings with adults. Even in compulsory drug treatment detention centres, there is little more than information provision of varying accuracy, and some counselling. The emphasis appears to be on 're-education', usually equated with admonitions to obey the law, discipline, physical activity and work.

Substance use among juvenile detainees

The use of alcohol and other drugs increases the likelihood of young people being detained simply for possession or use of such substances. Regular and heavy use of alcohol and other drugs also increases the likelihood of young people being involved in acquisitive crime, including drug dealing, to cover the cost of their substance use. While the use of illicit drugs can be one of the symptoms of conduct disorder, longitudinal studies have shown that young people tend to be involved in criminal activity prior to the onset of illicit drug use (Fergusson, Swain-Campbell and Horwood 2002). The presence of other mental health disorders also increases the likelihood of substance use and vulnerability to detention.

A strong association between substance use and involvement in delinquent or criminal activity is firmly established in the literature (McBride *et al.* 1999; Elliott, Huizinga and Ageton 1985; Nurco, Kinlock and Balter 1993; Dembo *et al.* 1994; Wong 2002). Longitudinal studies have shown that in a cohort of repeat offenders the onset of substance use can be part of a developmental trajectory to their offending behaviour (Nurco, Kinlock and Balter 1993; Fergusson, Swain-Campbell and Horwood 2002). It has also been found that the earlier drug use is established the greater its likelihood of continuing and leading into criminal activity (Fergusson and Horwood 1996).

In surveys of young people in detention in Australia conducted in the past decade, patterns of alcohol and other drug use were markedly different from those of their age peers in the Australian community and more like those of young people in Australian residential alcohol and other drug treatment services (Howard and Zibert 1990; Hando, Howard and Zibert 1997; Spooner, Mattick and Noffs 2000). Their average age of initiation to illicit drugs was significantly lower than the population average, being 12.3 years for cannabis compared with 18.4 years in the 1998 National Household Survey, and 14.7 years compared with 21.7 years for heroin (Johnson 2001). Consistent with these findings was the high level of injecting drug use, with more than a third of the sample reporting ever having injected a drug compared with less than 1 per cent of their same-age peers in the community (AIHW 1999).

Surveys of detained young people detail significant psychiatric morbidity in addition to substance use disorders (Scott, Snowden and Libby 2002), with more than half in a US sample meeting criteria for a mental disorder in the past year. This was most commonly attention deficit hyperactivity disorder or conduct disorders (47.9 per cent), with major depression accounting for less than 5 per cent of all disorders (Garland *et al.* 2001). A later, randomly selected and stratified sample of arrested and newly detained youth reported that 14 per cent of females and 11 per cent of males have had both a major mental disorder (psychosis, manic episode or major depressive episode) and a substance use disorder (Abram *et al.* 2003). Similar rates have been reported in Belgium (Vermeiren *et al.* 2004).

Findings such as these highlight the need for appropriate assessment and intervention in mental health, alcohol and other drug and juvenile justice programmes to interrupt the trajectory through the three systems.

Young people, sex and juvenile detention

In association with social marginalisation and drug related risk taking, young people in detention are highly vulnerable to the acquisition and transmission of sexually transmitted infections (STIs) (Eng and Butler 1997), with more limited access to health care (Glaser and Greifinger 1993). Young people in detention can be exposed to greater risk of sexual assault and exposure to blood-borne viruses and other sexually transmitted diseases as a result of consensual and non-consensual sexual activity with other detainees and/or staff, drug use, and tattooing (Helms and Hirbour 2004). This risk is further enhanced where the young person is detained in contexts that permit contact with adults.

US monitoring studies have indicated that rates of gonorrhoea among young detainees are 152 times greater among males and 42 times greater among females than among age matched counterparts in the general population (Shafer et al. 1993). In a later and larger US study, the vast majority of young men in detention testing positive for gonorrhoea did not report symptoms, which makes treatment unlikely without screening in juvenile detention facilities (Mertz et al. 2002). Particular populations in juvenile detention, such as African-American young people, may be at particular risk, with a study in southern USA reporting that those with involvement in the juvenile justice system had significantly higher rates of ever having gonorrhoea, chlamydia or trichomoniasis and were almost three times as likely to report using alcohol and drugs during their last sexual experience than their peers not in contact with juvenile justice (Crosby et al. 2003).

Detained young people also have elevated exposure to drug, sex and tattoo/body piercing related risk factors for HIV (Braithwaite et al. 2001). A recent study among clients of an HIV testing centre in Brazil identified juvenile detention as an independent predictor of subsequent HIV infection (Barcellos, Fuchs and Fuchs 2003). A Spanish study of detained young people reported that 2 per cent screened positive for HIV, 5.2 per cent for hepatitis C, but less than 1 per cent for syphilis (Olivan 2001). A later US study of incarcerated young people reported that 2 per cent of those tested were hepatitis C positive, which is higher than the general paediatric population (Murray et al. 2003).

Studies in the USA and Australia have shown that knowledge of HIV and hepatitis C is low among detained young people (Copeland, Howard and Fleischmann 1998), and lower among African-American compared with Caucasian samples (Canterbury et al. 1998). A UNICEF summary report from a series of Rapid Assessment and Response (RAR) studies on HIV/AIDS among especially vulnerable young people in South Eastern Europe noted that juvenile detainees tended not to have sufficient information on STIs and that most of the serious criminal acts were committed under the influence of drugs or committed to obtain funds to purchase drugs (Wong 2002). Wong found that of the sexually active juvenile offenders in her study in the Former Yugoslav Republic of Macedonia, 50 per cent shared injecting equipment, only 20 per cent reported 'always using a condom' during sex, and only 24 per cent had been tested for HIV.

In addition to addressing knowledge deficits, studies recommend that programmes to reduce HIV-related risk among young people in detention should address impulsivity (Devieux *et al.* 2002). A recent US survey also concluded that the public health system should provide HIV-related programming for young people in detention as many will have missed school-based interventions. Programmes should aim to intervene in the 10–13 years age group where risk is lowest, and specialist work is needed with girls, among injecting drug users, for those involved in sex work (Teplin *et al.* 2003) and for men who have sex with men.

In some developing countries, young people, often between the ages of 14 and 16 years, may be placed with older substance users in compulsory treatment centres where the HIV prevalence among the population can reach 70 per cent, or higher, with similar rates for hepatitis C. In these circumstances, programming must extend beyond information provision to encompass the protection of detainees from the risk of transmission of all blood-borne infections.

Theoretical models of the link between juvenile crime and substance use

Three main theoretical models have attempted to explain the nature of the relationship between juvenile crime and substance use. The first asserts that substance use causes crime (e.g. Gropper 1984; Nurco, Kinlock and Balter 1993), and is a model of the relationship that is popular in the minds of the general public. It assumes that illicit drug users generate the necessary income to support their substance use via crime (Ball *et al.* 1981) and/or that the psycho-pharmacological effects of drugs increase the users' propensity to commit crime, especially violent crime (White, Pandina and LaGrange 1987). Studies report that annual rates of delinquent offending increase directly with more serious drug involvement (Johnson *et al.* 1991), and Dembo and colleagues (1994) found that delinquent behaviour increases following involvement in illicit drug use, and that arrests for drug and property offences decline with decreasing frequency of drug use.

The second model of the relationship between juvenile crime and substance use argues that crime leads to substance use. According to this hypothesis, involvement in delinquency provides the context, the reference group, and definitions of the situation that are conducive to subsequent involvement with drugs (Bachman, O'Malley and Johnston 1978; Huizinga, Menard and Elliott 1989). Longitudinal studies of boys have reported that previous involvement in property offences increases the risk of the onset of illegal substance use (van Kammen and Loeber 1994). Fergusson, Swain-Campbell and Horwood (2002) have reported on the role of deviant peers in mediating the relationship between violent and property crime, and substance use, particularly among younger adolescents.

A third perspective is the 'common cause' model, which asserts that there is no causal link between substance use and crime but that the association is a spurious one born of similar aetiologies (e.g. Collins 1981; Jessor and Jessor 1977). Drug usage and delinquency are believed to cluster together as a result of experimentation with a wide range of behaviours in the teenage years. This problem behaviour syndrome or generality of deviance hypothesis (Donovan and Jessor 1985) is still open to question as different problem behaviours tend to follow different developmental paths; for example, delinquency peaks at ages 15–17 and then declines whereas poly-drug use increases into young adulthood (Elliott, Huizinga and Menard 1989).

In summary, a number of different perspectives exist concerning the relationship between juvenile crime and substance use. No studies have demonstrated a clear causal linkage, and it may be concluded that there are multiple pathways to the escalation of substance use and delinquent behaviour. Most of the principal variables act in association with one another rather than in a direct causal manner (Farrell 1993). There are, however, theoretically and clinically useful models of young people's substance use that are appropriate to the juvenile justice setting.

Programmatic implications

When it comes to promoting the health of young people in detention and, in particular, reducing drug- and sex-related risks, a number of options suggest themselves. In addition to expanding the means of diverting young people from custodial sentences by broadening the range of community-located interventions and services, there are a number of harm reduction responses that might be considered. These include risk reduction education (e.g. on the safer use of injecting equipment, sex and relationships education); hepatitis B vaccination; voluntary counselling and testing for sexually transmitted and blood-borne infections; the segregation from adults and more violent juvenile offenders and detainees; and drug dependence treatment in detention settings.

More controversial responses, particularly for young people, include condom distribution; the provision of sterile injecting equipment; and opioid substitution treatment such as methadone. In addition to any restrictions pertaining to age and minority status, where the majority of young people in detention are not injecting drug users the provision of injecting equipment and substitution treatment may be seen to entrench young people in a drug using culture and expose them to greater risk of dependency following their return to the community. However, there is little evidence to support such a view.

Among young people in refugee camps and in transitional and developing countries, there is an enhanced risk of being exposed to injecting drug use and sexual violence due to the stress of migration, and economic and social poverty. Models such as 'Triangular Clinics' in Iran offer promising approaches of good practice in the comprehensive and integrated management of HIV, sexually transmitted infections and drug use. Such an approach has been used in community settings and with detained populations in that country. The clinic provides a range of harm reduction services such as condoms, injecting equipment and methadone, HIV testing and counselling, prevention and treatment of sexually transmitted infections, referral to a range of community medical and social services, physical and psychological health services, social support and counselling and linkage to other non-government and government health and welfare services (WHO 2004).

While there is not strong evidence for improved treatment outcomes from mandated treatment, studies have demonstrated that pre-treatment arrests are negatively correlated with treatment completion among young people and that mandated entry into therapeutic communities is related to completion of the programme for all age levels (Catalano *et al.* 1990–1991). It has also been argued that mandated treatment can provide a young person with an excuse for being in treatment and provides an opportunity for trained, empathic staff to develop motivation for change (Howard 1994). The settings for and style of mandated treatment are, however, of considerable importance. While youth drug courts, in which offenders plead guilty to their offences and are involved in a wide range of mandated interventions, have shown some success in the USA and in Australia (Eardley *et al.* 2004), the US model of juvenile 'boot camps' is considerably less effective than the public believe, with extremely disappointing recidivism rates (Tyler, Darville and Stalnaker 2001).

Consistent with recommendations for juvenile justice generally, diversion from the juvenile corrections system appears to be the most promising method of intervention (Whitehead and Lab 1989). Young people who do not attract a custodial sentence should be referred to a comprehensive, non-residential treatment service and, where the circumstances are appropriate, with the possibility of legal sanctions for non-compliance. Such programmes should be conducted utilising the same broad principles as those in correctional settings.

Where this is not possible, upon entry to the juvenile justice system a young person should be appropriately assessed for substance use and related problems and the associated problems of family disruption, educational/employment problems, psychopathology, HIV risk taking behaviours, sexually transmitted infections, health and social functioning. Where substance use is identified, recommendation for intervention should be integrated into the appropriate justice system response, preferably diversion to community programmes which offer individual, group, family and community-wide programmatic interventions relevant to the areas identified in the assessment. For effectiveness, interventions should be provided by a variety of specialist services, linked by a coherent treatment plan.

For young people detained in custody and who are not currently involved in substance use, the promotion of health, life skills and appropriate role models may be of benefit (Rhodes and Jason 1988). Tackling the risk factors linked to poor social bonding and high levels of intra-personal distress is also essential. Additional primary prevention measures include parent education, especially improved parenting skills (Silverman and Silverman 1987) and community development.

For young people with a brief custodial sentence who have identified substance use-related difficulties, programmatic support should be initiated immediately upon entry to prepare the detainee for release with the development of effective links to a range of community-located services to support any change and provide necessary follow-up.

Randomised controlled trials provide minimal support for the superior effectiveness of any one treatment model for substance use disorders/problems among young people (Terry et al. 2000). Two therapeutic models, however – family therapy and skills training – show strong promise across multiple settings and populations. Integrative models, such as multi-systemic family therapy are the most promising family-based interventions (Liddle and Rowe 2002). Multi-systemic family therapy offers a comprehensive, family- and community-based treatment approach embedded within the family preservation model. It has recently shown promise in reducing drug-related delinquency behaviours including arrests, criminal offences and number of weeks in juvenile justice during follow-up (Henggeler et al. 1991).

These complex models, however, may not transport as effectively into treatment services (Henggeler, Pickrel and Brondino 1999). Similar models, such as multi-dimensional family therapy in residential or community settings, may also offer promising approaches (Liddle and Hogue 2000).

Programmatic responses such as these are, however, long term and resource intensive, and may be beyond the capacity of some developing, transitional and resource poor settings. Briefer, low cost cognitive-behavioural models of relapse prevention that include assertiveness training, communication skills, anger management, problem solving and techniques to cope with craving and high risk situations also show significant promise among this group (Catalano et al. 1990–1991; Dennis et al. 2004).

The cultural and social needs of sub-populations of young people in detention, such as girls, indigenous youth and those from other cultural and linguistic backgrounds, should be incorporated into any treatment strategy. This is especially important in the pre-release phase of work where introduction to community resources, referral to specialist services, and the identification of appropriate social supports is effected.

Conclusions

Diverting as many young people as possible from custodial environments should be a number one priority, given evidence that detention for minor offences such as the possession and use of illegal drugs does little to protect the community once the young person is released, or to protect the health and other rights of young people while in custodial settings. Young people in detention are a highly vulnerable group for substance use disorders, sexual abuse, blood-borne infections, STIs and mental health disorders.

There have been a wide range of social and legal responses to young people's substance use and crime, with wide ranging implications for personal, family and community cost. The juvenile justice system expects a reduction in offending rates, young offenders have a right to the full range of substance use, sexual health and mental health services, and governments demand cost effective services (Bailey 1999).

In order to secure such goals, future forms of service delivery should be developmentally appropriate; include thorough and standardised assessment; address structural determinants of substance use, sexual vulnerability and offending such as poverty, housing and educational opportunities; offer efficacious and ethical treatments; increase the competency of families and carers; and promote the prosocial development of young offenders (Bailey 1999). The juvenile justice system should also be accountable for clinical outcomes and ensure quality assurance mechanisms are in place to ensure a co-ordinated multi-agency response and continuity of care both within detention and in the community.

References

Abram, K., Teplin, L.A., McClelland, G.M. and Dulcan, M.K. (2003) 'Comorbid psychiatric disorders in youth in juvenile detention', *Archives of General Psychiatry*, 60: 1097–108.

American Bar Association (ABA) and the National Bar Association (2001) *Justice by Gender*, Chicago: ABA.

Australian Institute of Health and Welfare (AIHW) (1999) *National Drug Strategy Household Survey, 1998* [computer file]. Canberra: Social Science Data Archives, The Australian National University.

Australian Institute of Health and Welfare (AIHW) (2003) *Australia's Young People: Their Health and Wellbeing*, AIHW Cat. No. PHE 50. Canberra: Australian Institute of Health and Welfare.

Bachman, J.G., O'Malley, P.M. and Johnston, L.D. (1978) *Youth in Transition:*

Adolescence to Adulthood, Change and Stability in the Lives of Young Men, Vol. VI, Ann Arbor, Michigan: Institute for Social Research, University of Michigan.

Bailey, S. (1999) 'The interface between mental health, criminal justice and forensic mental health services for children and adolescents', *Current Opinion in Psychiatry*, 12(4): 425–32.

Ball, A.L., Rana, S. and Dehne, K.L. (1998) 'HIV prevention among injecting drug users: responses in developing and transitional countries', *Public Health Reports*, 113(Supp. 1): 170–81.

Ball, J.C., Rosen, L., Flueck, J.A. and Nurco, D.N. (1981) 'The criminality of heroin addicts when addicted and when off opiates', in J.A. Inciardi (ed.), *The Drugs–Crime Connection*, California: Sage.

Barcellos, N.T., Fuchs, D.S. and Fuchs, F.D. (2003) 'Prevalence and risk factors for HIV infection in individuals testing for HIV at counselling centers in Brazil', *Sexually Transmitted Diseases*, 30: 166–73.

Beale, S.S. (2003) 'Still tough on crime? Prospects for restorative justice in the United States', *Utah Law Review*, 1: 413–37.

Braithwaite, R., Robillard, A., Woodring, T., Stephens, S. and Kimberly, J.A. (2001) 'Tattooing and body piercing among adolescent detainees: relationship to alcohol and other drug use', *Journal of Substance Abuse*, 13: 5–16.

Canterbury, R.J., Clavet, G.J., McGarvey, E.L. and Koopman, C. (1998) 'HIV risk-related attitudes and behaviours of incarcerated adolescents: implications for public school students', *The High School Journal*, 82: 1–10.

Catalano, R.F., Hawkins, J.D., Wells, E.A. and Miller, J. (1990–1991) 'Evaluation of the effectiveness of adolescent drug abuse treatment, assessment of risks for relapse, and promising approaches for relapse prevention', *International Journal of the Addictions*, 25(9A and 10A): 1085–140.

Collins, J.J. (1981) *Drinking and Crime*, New York: Guilford.

Copeland, J., Howard, J. and Fleischmann, S. (1998) 'Gender, HIV knowledge and risk-taking behaviour among substance using adolescents in custody in New South Wales', *Journal of Substance Misuse*, 3: 206–12.

Crosby, R.A., DiClemente, R.J., Wingwood, G., Rose, E. and Levine, D. (2003) 'Adjudication history and African American adolescents' risk for acquiring sexually transmitted diseases: an exploratory analysis', *Sexually Transmitted Diseases*, 30: 634–8.

Dembo, R., Williams, L., Fagan, J. and Schmeidler, J. (1994) 'Development and assessment of a classification of high risk youth', *Journal of Drug Issues*, 24: 25–53.

Dennis, M., Godley, S.H., Diamond, G., Tims, F.M., Babor, T., Donaldson, J.H., Titus, J.C., Kamner, Y., Webb, C., Hamilton, N. and Funk, R. (2004) 'The Cannabis Youth Treatment (CYT) study: main findings from two randomized trials', *Journal of Substance Abuse Treatment*, 27: 197–213.

Devieux, J., Malow, R., Stein, J.A., Jennings, T.E., Lucenko, B.A., Averhart, C. and Kalichman, S. (2002) 'Impulsivity and HIV risk among adjudicated alcohol and other drug abusing adolescent offenders', *AIDS Education and Prevention*, 14(Supp. B): 24–35.

Donovan, J.E. and Jessor, R. (1985) 'Structure of problem behavior in adolescence and young adulthood', *Journal of Consulting and Clinical Psychology*, 53: 890–904.

Eardley, T., McNab, J., Fisher, K. and Kozlia, S. (2004) *Evaluation of the New South*

Wales Youth Drug Court Pilot Program, Sydney: Social Policy Research Centre, University of New South Wales Evaluation Consortium.

Elliott, D.S., Huizinga, D. and Ageton, S.S. (1985) *Explaining Delinquency and Drug Use*, California: Sage.

Elliott, D.S., Huizinga, D.M. and Menard, S. (1989) *Multiple Problem Youth: Delinquency, Substance Use and Mental Health Problems*, New York: Springer-Verlag.

Eng, T.R. and Butler, W.T. (eds) (1997) *The Hidden Epidemic: Confronting Sexually Transmitted Diseases*, Washington, DC: National Academy Press.

Farrell, A. (1993) 'Risk factors for drug use in urban adolescents: a three-wave longitudinal study', *Journal of Drug Issues*, 23(3): 443–62.

Feld, B.C. (2003) 'Race, politics, and juvenile justice: the Warren court and the conservative "backlash"', *Minnesota Law Review*, 87: 1447–577.

Fergusson, D.M. and Horwood, L.J. (1996) 'The role of adolescent peer affiliations in the continuity between childhood behavioural adjustment and juvenile offending', *Journal of Abnormal Child Psychology*, 24: 205–21.

Fergusson, D.M., Swain-Campbell, N.R. and Horwood, L.J. (2002) 'Deviant peer affiliations, crime and substance use: a fixed effects regression analysis', *Journal of Abnormal Child Psychology*, 30: 419–30.

Garland, A.E., Hough, R.L., McCabe, K.M., Yeh, M., Wood, P.A. and Aarons, G.A. (2001) 'Prevalence of psychiatric disorders in youths across five sectors of care', *Journal of the American Academy of Child and Adolescent Psychiatry*, 40: 409–18.

Glaser, J.B. and Greifinger, R.B. (1993) 'Correctional health care: a public health opportunity', *Annals of Internal Medicine*, 118: 139–45.

Gropper, B.A. (1984) *Probing the Links Between Drugs and Crime*, *National Institute of Justice Reports*, Washington, DC: National Institute of Justice.

Hando, J., Howard, J. and Zibert, E. (1997) 'Risky drug practices and treatment needs of youth detained in New South Wales Juvenile Justice Centre', *Drug and Alcohol Review*, 16: 137–45.

Helms, J.L. and Hirbour, C.A. (2004) 'HIV and juvenile delinquency', *American Journal of Forensic Psychology*, 22: 57–71.

Henggeler, S.W., Borduin, C.M., Melton, G.B., Mann, B.J., Smith, L., Hall, J.A., Cone, L. and Fucci, B.R. (1991) 'Effects of multisystemic therapy on drug use and abuse in serious and chronic juvenile offenders: a progress report from two outcome studies', *Family Dynamics of Addiction Quarterly*, 1: 40–51.

Henggeler, S.W., Pickrel, S.G. and Brondino, M.J. (1999) 'Multisystemic treatment of substance-abusing and dependent delinquents: outcomes, treatment fidelity and transportability', *Mental Health Services Research*, 1: 171–84.

Howard, J. (1994) 'Irrelevant, unapproachable or boring: treatment issues for drug-using youth', in J. Ross (ed.), *Health For All? Social Justice Issues in the Alcohol and Other Drugs Field*, Proceedings from the Sixth National Drug and Alcohol Research Centre Annual Symposium, December 1993. Sydney: NDARC Monograph Number 21: 92–119.

Howard, J. and Zibert, E. (1990) 'Curious, bored and wanting to feel good: the drug use of detained young offenders', *Drug and Alcohol Review*, 9: 225–31.

Huizinga, D.H., Menard, S. and Elliott, D.S. (1989) 'Delinquency and drug use: temporal developmental patterns', *Justice Quarterly*, 6: 419–55.

Human Rights Watch (1998) *Abandoned to the State: Cruelty and Neglect in Russian Orphanages*, New York: Human Rights Watch. Online. Available HTTP: <http://www.hrw.org/reports98/russia2/> (accessed August 2004).

Human Rights Watch (2001) *Easy Targets: Violence Against Children Worldwide*, New York: Human Rights Watch. Online. Available HTTP: http://www.hrw.org/reports/2001/children (accessed August 2004).

Human Rights Watch (2004) *Children's Rights: Juvenile Justice*, New York: Human Rights Watch. Online. Available HTTP: <http://www.hrw.org/children/justice.htm> (accessed January 2005).

Jessor, R. and Jessor, S. (1977) *Problem Behavior and Psychosocial Development: A Longitudinal Study of Youth*, New York: Academic Press.

Johnson, B.D., Wish, E.D., Schmeidler, J. and Huizinga, D. (1991) 'Concentration of delinquent offending: serious drug involvement and high delinquency rates', *Journal of Drug Issues*, 21: 205–29.

Johnson, D. (2001) 'Age of illicit drug initiation', *Trends and Issues in Crime and Criminal Justice, No. 201*, Canberra: Australian Institute of Criminology.

Lederman, C.S., Dakof, G.A., Larrea, M.A. and Li, H. (2004) 'Characteristics of adolescent girls in detention', *International Journal of Law and Psychiatry*, 27: 321–37.

Liddle, H.A. and Hogue, A. (2000) 'A family-based ecological preventive intervention for antisocial behavior in high-risk adolescents', *Journal of Family and Marital Therapy*, 26: 265–80.

Liddle, H.A. and Rowe, C.L. (2002) 'Adolescent drug abuse: making the case for a developmental-contextual, family-based intervention', in D.W. Brook and H.I. Spitz (eds), *The Group Psychotherapy of Substance Abuse* (pp. 275–80), Washington, DC: American Psychiatric Press.

McBride, D.E., VanderWaal, C.J., Terry, Y.M. and VanBuren, H. (1999) *Breaking the Cycle of Drug Use Among Juvenile Offenders*, Final Technical Report: National Institute of Justice. Web only document. Online. Available HTTP: <http://www.ncjrs.org/pdffiles1/nij/179273.pdf>

Mertz, K.J., Voigt, R.A., Hutchins, K., Levine, W.C. and the Jail STD Monitoring Group (2002) 'Findings from STD screening of adolescents and adults entering corrections facilities: implications for STD control strategies', *Sexually Transmitted Diseases*, 29: 834–9.

Murray, K.F., Richardson, L.P., Morishima, C., Owens, J. and Gretch, D.R. (2003) 'Prevalence of hepatitis C virus infection and risk factors in an incarcerated juvenile population: a pilot study', *Pediatrics*, 111: 153–7.

Nurco, D.N., Kinlock, T. and Balter, M.B. (1993) 'The severity of preaddiction criminal behavior among urban male narcotic addicts and two nonaddicted control groups', *Journal of Research in Crime and Delinquency*, 30(3): 293–316.

Office of the High Commissioner for Human Rights (1985) *United Nations Standard Minimum Rules for the Administration of Juvenile Justice ('The Beijing Rules')*. Online. Available HTTP: <http://www.unhchr.ch/html/menu3/b/h_comp48.htm>

Olivan, G. (2001) 'The health profile of Spanish incarcerated delinquent youths', *Journal of Adolescent Health*, 29: 384.

Physicians for Human Rights (n.d.) *Girls in the System*, Cambridge MA: Physicians for Human Rights. Online. Available HTTP: http://www.phrusa.org/campaigns/juv_justice/girls.html (accessed July 2004).

Reitsma-Street, M. (1999) 'Justice for Canadian girls: a 1990s update', *Canadian Journal of Criminology*, 41: 335–63.

Rhodes, J. and Jason, L. (1988) *Preventing Substance Abuse Among Children and Adolescents*, New York: Pergamon.

Scott, M.A., Snowden, L. and Libby, A.M. (2002) 'From mental health to juvenile justice: what factors predict this transition?' *Journal of Child and Family Studies*, 11: 299–311.

Shafer, M.A., Hilton, J.F., Ekstrand, M., Keogh, J., Gee, L., DiGiorgio-Haag, L., Shalwitz, J. and Schachter, J. (1993) 'Relationship between drug use and sexual behaviours and the occurrence of sexually transmitted diseases among high risk male youth', *Sexually Transmitted Diseases*, 20: 307–13.

Silverman, W. and Silverman, M. (1987) 'Using demographic data in a primary prevention substance abuse program for teenagers and parents', *Psychology of Addictive Behaviors*, 1: 163–72.

Spooner, C., Mattick, R.P. and Noffs, W. (2000) 'A study of the patterns and correlates of substance use among adolescents applying for drug treatment', *Australian and New Zealand Journal of Public Health*, 24: 492–502.

Teplin, L.A., Mericle, A.A., McClelland, G.M. and Abram, K. (2003) 'HIV and AIDS risk behaviours in juvenile detainees: implications for public health policy', *American Journal of Public Health*, 93: 906–12.

Terry, Y.M., VanderWaal, C.J., McBride, D.C. and Van Buren, H. (2000) 'Provision of drug treatment services in the juvenile justice system: a system reform', *Journal of Behavioral Health Services and Research*, 27: 194–214.

Tyler, J., Darville, R. and Stalnaker, K. (2001) 'Juvenile boot camps: a descriptive analysis of program diversity and effectiveness', *Social Science Journal*, 38: 445–60.

UNICEF (n.d.) 'Juvenile justice.' Online. Available HTTP: <http://www.unicef.org/protection/index_juveniljustice.html>

van Kammen, W.B. and Loeber, R. (1994) 'Are fluctuations in delinquent activities related to the onset and offset in juvenile illegal drug use and drug dealing?' *Journal of Drug Issues*, 24: 9–24.

Vermeiren, R., Jones, S.M., Ruchkin, V., Deboutte, D. and Schwab-Stone, M. (2004) 'Juvenile arrest: a cross-cultural comparison', *Journal of Child Psychology and Psychiatry*, 45: 567–76.

White, H.R., Pandina, R.J. and LaGrange, R.L. (1987) 'Longitudinal predictors of serious substance use and delinquency', *Criminology*, 25: 715–40.

Whitehead, J.T. and Lab, S.P. (1989) 'A meta-analysis of juvenile correctional treatment', *Journal of Research in Crime and Delinquency*, 26: 276–95.

Wong, E. (2002) *Rapid Assessment and Response on HIV/AIDS among Especially Vulnerable Young People in South Eastern Europe*, Balkans: UNICEF.

World Health Organization (2004) *Best Practice in HIV/AIDS Prevention and Care for Injecting Drug Abusers: The Triangular Clinic and Kermanshah, Islamic Republic of Iran*, Cairo: WHO Regional Office for the Eastern Mediterranean.

Chapter 13

Sex, drugs and indigenous young people

Sherry Saggers, Dennis Gray and Phillipa Strempel

Throughout the world, changing social and cultural factors shape the developing identities of young people and frame how behaviours such as sexual activity and substance use will be viewed (Figueroa, Infante and Senna 2000; Sercombe 1997). The demonising of young people (Pearson 1983) has meant that much of what has been said and written of sex and drug use and young people is overwhelmingly negative, focusing on the adverse health and social effects of these behaviours rather than on more positive features (Aggleton, Ball and Mane 2000). This emphasis on the pathological means that we still know relatively little about normal sexual development and drug use among young people in general, and indigenous young people in particular.

Indigenous peoples – the original inhabitants of the countries considered in this chapter – are heterogeneous and geographically widespread. Nevertheless, they share certain characteristics including their pre-existence in a place prior to the arrival of another population; political subordination within the nation-state; self-identification as indigenous people; and cultural distinctiveness from the rest of the state's population (Burger 1987; Kingsbury 1995; United Nations Commission on Human Rights 1994). Even within first world countries, indigenous minorities are not homogeneous. Particularly in the USA, Canada and Australia, there is considerable social and cultural variation. Nevertheless, with the inclusion of the indigenous people of New Zealand, these peoples do share a common history of colonialism, dispossession and exclusion and for these reasons these indigenous minority peoples of settler colonial societies are the focus of this chapter.

Indigenous peoples in Europe, Asia and Latin America share many of the characteristics of the peoples discussed here, with respect to licit and illicit drug use, and the consequences of sexual activities on their lives. There is a growing literature on alcohol use among the Saami of Europe (Larsen and Saglie 1996), opiate use in many Asian countries (Cherry 2002), and stimulant and hallucinogen use in Latin American communities (Schultes 1990), for example. And there is also research on a burgeoning sex industry exploiting indigenous young people in parts of Asia, including hill tribe communities such as the Hmong in northern Thailand, where the destruction of traditional economies has forced indigenous young women (and some young men) into prostitution and exposed them and their communities to injecting drug use and HIV (Symonds 1998). However, space and the cultural diversity among indigenous peoples of Australia, Canada, the USA and New Zealand alone has necessitated the restriction of focus in this chapter.

It is not simply cultural heterogeneity which influences sexual activity and drug use. The social circumstances of indigenous young people may be more important for their health status than their cultural differences. Gender, sexuality, age, educational and occupational status, income, and family organisation all structure the way in which indigenous young people engage with the wider societies in which they live, and may significantly influence their biological and social development, including sexual and substance use behaviours. Determining the relative importance of these social factors is complex (Loxley et al. 2003).

Patterns of sexual activity and substance use

Reviewing indigenous sexual activity and drug use is limited by the wide variation in the peoples under consideration, and the small number of relevant studies and methodological variation between them, inhibiting direct comparisons or extrapolation to larger populations. This is particularly the case with respect to sexual activity. Nevertheless, some generalisations are possible.

Sexual activity and its health consequences

Internationally there is evidence of young people having sex earlier, and more of them becoming sexually active with more partners than young people in the past (Pool et al. 1999; Johnson et al. 1994). The adverse health consequences of these trends include sexually transmitted infections and early pregnancies. Younger mothers are more likely to experience complications while giving birth, to have low birth-weight babies, and to have babies who die in their infancy (AIHW 2003; Brady 1991). Teenage parenthood is associated with socio-economic disadvantage throughout the life of an individual and intergenerationally (Morris, Warren and Aral 1993).

Indigenous young people are more likely to be sexually active and at an earlier age than their non-indigenous counterparts (Blum et al. 1992; Brady 1991; Chewning et al. 2001; Fenwicke and Purdie 2000; Lynskey and Fergusson 1993; Social Exclusion Unit 1999). In New Zealand, for instance, a study of the sexual activity of high school students showed that Māori students were nearly three times more likely to have had sex than their non-Māori counterparts. Young Māori women who reported having sex were four times more likely to report having more than five partners than non-Māori respondents, and three times as likely to report having sex before they were 12. Young Māori men were also likely to report more sex partners, and earlier sex than their non-Māori counterparts (Fenwicke and Purdie 2000).

Use of contraception is lower among some indigenous young people and the consequences of early, unprotected sexual activity among young people include higher rates of pregnancy and childbirth than among the general population (Blum *et al.* 1992; Brady 1991; AIHW 2003). In Australia, for instance, indigenous women begin bearing children at an earlier age than their non-indigenous counterparts. Although the percentage was declining, in the period 1994–1996, almost a quarter of indigenous mothers were teenagers – nearly five times the proportion among non-indigenous mothers (Day, Sullivan and Lancaster 1999). In part, these patterns relate to the positive value of children and child-bearing in indigenous communities, and young women are more likely to express a desire to have children early (Blum *et al.* 1992).

Indigenous young women are also more likely to be hospitalised for complications arising from pregnancy and childbirth, than their non-indigenous counterparts. In New Zealand, for instance, in 1994, most hospitalisations of females aged 12–25 years were for complications of pregnancy and childbirth, and the rate among Māori was five times that for non-Māori (Statistics New Zealand 1998: 93, 96). Similar patterns are apparent in Australia (AIHW 2003: 339–40).

Sexually transmitted infections are much more common among indigenous young people than amongst the general populations in all of the countries discussed here. For instance, in Canada, sex- and age-specific rates of genital chlamydia are higher among First Nations populations than Canadians generally, in all categories, but the largest difference by far is in the 15 to 19 years age group. If left untreated, genital chlamydia can result in pelvic inflammatory disease, increased risk of ectopic pregnancy and infertility (Health Canada 2001). While it is important to avoid alarmist accounts of these infections, they do indicate the potential sexual exploitation of sometimes very young people. Until recently, talking publicly about the sexual abuse of children in most countries was rare, but indigenous peoples themselves are demanding investigation of what is seen as a blight on whole communities.

It is evident that earlier sexual activity, lower contraception use, earlier child bearing and complications arising from this among indigenous young people do have serious health and social consequences for these young people. But we still know relatively little about their knowledge of sexual health issues and if they share the concerns of health professionals and others. Young people's sexuality has to be seen in the broader social and cultural context in which sexual activity and pregnancy may be positively viewed as signalling adult status, and where alternative avenues of status, such as education and employment, may be limited. On the other hand, some young people experience unwanted sexual attention, because of the widespread use of alcohol and other drugs in many communities. All of these factors mean that non-judgemental and culturally sensitive approaches to young people's sexual health are necessary.

Drug use

Despite the moral panics associated with drug use by indigenous people and a higher prevalence of drug use among them than in non-indigenous populations, the majority of people use drugs without problems. This point has been made with regard to alcohol use among indigenous people in Australia, New Zealand and Canada (Durie 2001; Saggers and Gray 1998) and the USA (Rice 1996). It is also evident with regard to other drugs in Australia (Australia, Department of Health and Family Services 1995). In fact, data from Australia, New Zealand and Canada show that fewer indigenous than non-indigenous people consume alcohol, but that those who do so consume it at higher levels (Durie 2001; Saggers and Gray 1998). However, substance use by a significant minority is having serious health and social consequences and indigenous peoples throughout the world have acknowledged the need to tackle the issue in a positive way (Durie 2001; Saggers and Gray 1998).

Drug use among young, primary school children does not appear to be ethnically patterned, at least in Australia (Dunne, Yeo and Keane 2000; Gray et al. 1997). It is only when young people enter secondary (high) school that increases in drug use with age occur, especially among indigenous young people (Forero et al. 1999; Gray et al. 1997). This pattern, with the exception of volatile substances, has also been shown in the USA (Beauvais 1992a, 1992b).

A study from Australia found that, among secondary students aged 12–17 years, the lifetime prevalence of alcohol use and the prevalence of regular drinking (three or more times in the previous month) were very similar between indigenous and non-indigenous students. However, as with the adult populations in all countries under consideration, hazardous drinking was twice as common among indigenous students (Forero et al. 1999: 298). Similar patterns have been reported among reservation Indian, non-reservation Indian, and Anglo (i.e. Americans of European descent) twelfth graders in the United States (Beauvais 1992a, 1992b), and Māori between the ages of 14 and 17 years (BRC Marketing and Social Research 2003: 6).

Tobacco smoking among indigenous young people has not attracted as much attention as alcohol and other drugs, but is potentially more serious. In Australia, tobacco is the single greatest cause of mortality among indigenous people and they currently smoke at around twice the rate of the non-indigenous population (Australia, Department of Health and Family

Services 1995). This difference is also reflected among secondary school students, among whom 31 per cent of indigenous students and 21 per cent of non-indigenous students reported smoking tobacco in the previous week (Forero et al.1999: 298). Again, these patterns are repeated in the USA, where Beauvais reported a similar pattern among students – at least with regard to lifetime prevalence of smoking (Beauvais 1992a) and in New Zealand where, in 1996, 31 per cent of Māori males and 41 per cent of Māori females aged 15–19 years reported smoking regularly compared to 18 per cent of both non-Māori males and females (Statistics New Zealand 1998: 89). Indigenous people are also likely to take up smoking earlier than their non-indigenous counterparts (Australia, Department of Health and Family Services 1995).

After alcohol and tobacco, cannabis is the drug that is most frequently consumed by indigenous school students. In the USA, among twelfth graders, Beauvais reported a lifetime prevalence of cannabis use among more than three-quarters of reservation Indians, 58 per cent among non-reservation Indians, and 38 per cent among Anglos. The 30-day prevalence among students was 33 per cent among reservation Indians, 21 per cent among non-reservation Indians, and 13 per cent among Anglos (Beauvais 1992b). In Australia, lifetime prevalence of cannabis use was reported by half of students compared to 36 per cent among non-students, and indigenous males and females were more likely to report weekly use of cannabis than non-indigenous males and females (Forero et al. 1999: 298). Earlier up-take and high and rising rates of cannabis use among Māori compared to non-Māori are also reported (New Zealand, Ministry of Health 1995; Durie 2001).

Inhalant use is common for both indigenous and non-indigenous students at some point in their lives. In the USA, among young people aged around 18 years, 20 per cent of reservation Indians, 15 per cent of non-reservation Indians, and 10 per cent of Anglos reported a lifetime prevalence of inhalant use (Beauvais 1992b). In Australia, the lifetime prevalence of indigenous and non-indigenous secondary students was surprisingly similar (33 per cent and 27 per cent respectively) (Forero et al. 1999: 298). In both countries, the use of inhalants declines with age as other substances become more accessible and affordable, and is more common in remote communities (Beauvais 1992b; Brady 1992).

Use of illicit drugs – such as hallucinogens, amphetamines and opioids – is less common but the pattern of higher use among indigenous students remains the same (Forero et al. 1999; Beauvais 1992b; Durie 2001). Injection of some of these drugs is even less common (Australia, Department of Health and Family Services 1995; Beauvais 1992b). Nevertheless, injecting is of concern, and appears to be increasing (Gray et al. 2001). In Australia, the median age at which injecting commenced was between 15 and 17 years (Gray et al. 2001; Larson, Shannon and Eldridge 1999; Shoobridge 1998). Evidence of widespread sharing of needles among indigenous people who inject drugs is also a major concern (Gray *et al.* 2001; Shoobridge 1998).

Indigenous young people, like their non-indigenous counterparts, are likely to be poly-drug users (Burns and Currie 1995; Gray *et al.* 2001). Not all drugs are equally problematic, from a health or community perspective, with indigenous communities in most countries highlighting the serious impacts of alcohol, solvent abuse and illicit drugs (Durie 2001; Saggers and Gray 1998). Interventions need to take this poly-drug use into account, together with communities' priorities.

Health consequences of substance use

Trying to determine the health impacts of substance use is complex, due to differences in measurements across countries. However, some patterns are apparent. In Australia, New Zealand and the USA, the leading causes of death among all young people are motor vehicle accidents, suicide and non-motor vehicle accidents. In all three countries, however, the rates among indigenous people are considerably higher than those among non-indigenous people (AIHW 2003: 333–5; Statistics New Zealand 1998: 82–5; IHS 2003: 67). In the USA, for example, the rate ratios are at least 2.4:1 and are at least equally elevated among indigenous people in Australia and New Zealand. As in the USA, in Australia and New Zealand these rates are also skewed towards males.

These leading causes of death among young people are not all alcohol- or other drug-related, but they do reflect the consequences of higher rates of hazardous or problem use among indigenous peoples. In the USA in 1994–96, the deaths attributable to 'alcoholism' were over ten times greater among Native Americans aged 15–24 years than among 'whites' (IHS 2003: 110). Estimates for Australia are that in 2001, among non-indigenous people aged 15–29 years, alcohol was a causal factor in around a third of all suicides (personal communication Tanya Chikriths, National Alcohol Indicators Project, National Drug Research Institute) and that these percentages are likely to be higher in indigenous people. Alcohol is similarly implicated in the other leading causes of death.

Substance use also contributes to higher levels of illness and social disruption for indigenous young people, their families and communities. Understanding how this happens requires more detailed analysis of the social determinants of health behaviours than is possible here.

Situating sex and drug use in social and cultural contexts

Having sex and using alcohol and other drugs are a normal part of life for many young people, and indigenous young people are no different from their non-indigenous peers in this respect. It is only when early sexual activity and substance use result in adverse health and social outcomes that such behaviours become problematic. Understanding why indigenous young people are more likely than their non-indigenous peers to experience adverse outcomes from these behaviours requires an examination of the social and cultural contexts of their lives.

Social determinants of health

Contemporary social models of health acknowledge the role of interconnected levels of social factors from the most broadly structural (such as the impact of colonisation); through social categories immediate to the individual (such as the influence of family and friends) and more distant (the impact of neighbourhood and community); to individual characteristics (including socio-economic circumstances and health behaviours) (Lynch 2000; Marmot and Wilkinson 1999; Kawachi 2000; Najman 2001).

The challenge has been to demonstrate the way in which social variables are causally related to health and illness. Socio-economic status, which combines income, education and occupation levels, is the most common means by which the health of individuals or groups has been measured. It is apparently not simply absolute deprivation which causes ill health, but inequalities in the distribution of material resources within countries that is also associated with poor health status (Keating and Hertzman 1999; Daniels, Kennedy and Kawachi 1999). This has important implications for many of the world's indigenous peoples who live in developed countries, but in conditions more similar to those in less developed nations (Saggers and Gray 1991, 1998).

Researchers of indigenous health in Australia, Canada, New Zealand and the USA have noted the disastrous consequences of colonialism on the health of people, and have shown how this is linked to social and economic marginalisation, institutional and personal racism, restricted access to health services, and higher levels of behavioural risk factors such as smoking and heavy drinking (Saggers and Gray 1991, 1998; Durie 1998, 2001; Stubben 1997). But these relationships are complex, and determining how aspects of the social environment make us physically sick has directed attention to the way in which social capital, or the depth and breadth of social connections in any community, helps to explain health outcomes (Kawachi, Kennedy and Glass 1999).

Individuals' experiences of the social world are also culturally mediated (Eckersley 2001; Durie 2001). Some suggest that the cultural qualities of contemporary social life, particularly those influencing family life, work and education, lead many young people to view the risks they face as 'personal and individual, rather than structural and collective' (Eckersley 2001: 66). Others believe cultural factors such as religious observance or adherence to cultural values protect individuals and groups against risky health behaviours, hence conferring health advantages (Durie 2001; Najman 2001; O'Nell and Mitchell 1996). In Australia, Canada, New Zealand and the USA, indigenous communities are drawing upon their traditional cultures to promote healthier living. For instance, traditional gatherings such as *pow-wows* in parts of the USA are being used as vehicles for health promotional messages about alcohol and other drugs (May and Moran 1995). The evidence, however, is ambiguous, and it may be that structural factors, social relationships, peer groups, family interactions, and individual adjustment explain most variation among indigenous young people (Young 1992).

While much illness is socially and culturally determined, some individuals maintain good health in spite of their social circumstances. Understanding the way in which individual health is compromised by risk factors, or enhanced through protective factors, has been important to the development of a coherent social model of health (Cashmore 2001; Loxley *et al.* 2003).

Social determinants of sexual behaviour

Trying to explain sexual behaviours is difficult, but it seems clear that these behaviours are linked to both broad social factors, and cultural factors specific to each group. Among many populations, low socio-economic status is associated with higher rates of sexual activity at younger ages (Morris, Warren and Aral 1993; Lynskey and Fergusson 1993; Social Exclusion Unit 1999). Indigenous young people the world over experience low socio-economic status because of their poor schooling and high rates of unemployment (Trewin and Madden 2003; Lynskey and Fergusson 1993). They are largely born into families whose members have themselves been excluded from education and employment and who struggle to provide the kind of guidance and supervision necessary to cope with the requirements of school and work, particularly when exacerbated by institutional and personal racism.

In traditionally oriented indigenous societies, transitions to adulthood involved rites of passage which gradually inculcated social and religious knowledge equipping young people to take their place in adult society. In indigenous Australia, for example, boys in Arnhem Land as young as 7 or 8 would begin ritual inductions into manhood which would continue through their adult lives (Brady 1991). Young women had fewer ceremonial rituals to celebrate their coming change of status, and this period was more likely to be marked by marriage and child-bearing and rearing. At around the age of 9 or 10, girls could be married and took up residence in their husband's household (Burbank 1988).

At this time, both young men and women were expected to contribute economically to their households, and behave as socially responsible adults.

This is quite different from the expectations for indigenous young people in most societies today. Many of them are excluded from the mainstream economy because of inadequate education and training, and even in remote areas, few are likely to participate in traditional hunting or other pursuits. Instead many find themselves with much unstructured time in which to hang around together in same-sex groups, taking on many of the beliefs, values and material possessions of Western young people (Brady 1991). It is this combination of much free time, and lack of meaningful access to educational and employment opportunities that may contribute to unsafe sex and early pregnancy.

Protective factors associated with indigenous young people's safer sex (measured in terms of abstention from intercourse and/or consistent use of birth control) have to do with family and friends, and education. Having peers who are perceived to have fewer risky behaviours, parents who are knowledgeable about sexual health and who monitor their activities, valuing education and achieving well at school, and believing oneself to be responsible for sexual health are all associated with safer sexual activity among American Indian young people from rural areas (Chewning *et al.* 2001). In this same study, self-esteem (which has frequently been cited as contributing to poor sexual health) and cultural-connectedness did not appear to be associated with the adolescents' sexual behaviour, reinforcing the notion that while cultural factors are important, they may not be as influential as broader structural factors.

Social determinants of substance use

The adverse health and social impacts of alcohol and other drug use among indigenous people have been attributed by many researchers to a broad range of long-standing social determinants (Coleman, Grant and Collins 2001; Durie 2001; Hunter 1993; Spooner, Hall and Lynskey 2001; Forero *et al.* 1999; Gray *et al.* 1996; Oetting, Beauvais and Edwards 1988), including experiences of colonialism, dispossession and continuing exclusion from wider economic and social life. The consequences of this history include low levels of school retention and participation in the workforce, compared to their counterparts in the general population (Saggers and Gray 1998; Gray and Saggers 2002; Durie 2001).

A number of studies link substance use problems among young indigenous people to these social indicators (Beauvais *et al.* 2002; Durie 2001; Forero *et al.* 1999; Comeau and Santin 1995). Two comprehensive national Australian surveys revealed that young people 15 and over who had completed at least year 12 were less likely to report that they smoked, than were those who had real employment (rather than work for social security entitlements) (in Loxley *et al.* 2003). A small study among young people in Western Australia found that children who were disaffected from school were 23 times more likely to be poly-drug users; and that older young people who were unemployed were 13.5 times more likely to be frequent poly-drug users than those who were employed, in training, or still at school (Gray *et al.* 1996).

Social relationships with families also have a significant impact on the drug use of young indigenous people. A number of studies among young American Indians, Native Alaskans, Native Canadians, Māori and Australians have demonstrated how they are more likely to have absent or ineffective parental role models, for reasons including the death of a parent (Blum *et al.* 1992), parental unemployment or conflict (Brady 1991; Oetting, Beauvais and Edwards 1988; Durie 2001), parental substance use (Davey and Dawes 1994; Oetting, Beauvais and Edwards 1988; Durie 2001), and low parental supervision (Forero *et al.* 1999). Conversely, strong family structures protect against sustained problematic substance use by young people (Durie 2001).

Peers, too, can either encourage a young person to take up harmful drinking and drug taking, or provide an environment where such behaviour is positively valued (Beauvais *et al.* 2002; Davey and Dawes 1994; Oetting, Beauvais and Edwards 1988). But we also need to understand how common this behaviour is among young people worldwide: 'Binge drinking among Māori youth as part of a socialising ritual is not a uniquely Māori experience; it has much in common with youth in other parts of the world' (Durie 2001: 34). One Australian study has shown that if a young person's friends use marijuana, they are 60–80 per cent more likely to use it as well (Larson *et al.* 1997). In the USA, too, young indigenous people who were heavy drug users were more likely to have friends who used and encouraged drug use (Beauvais 1992c). These peers are less likely than non-indigenous young people to see substance use as primarily adolescent behaviour which is gradually brought under control as a young person takes on more adult roles – such as further education, training and employment (Davey and Dawes 1994).

In some circumstances, however, substance use may become an important part of indigenous cultural identity, as a response to economic and political marginalisation (Blum *et al.* 1992; Brady 1991; Durie 2001). According to one young indigenous Australian:

> We all thought school sucks because we got cousins and brothers sitting around on the dole 'cause they can't find no work. So we knew our turn is comin' up when we leave, so we get used to get stoned all the time.
>
> (Davey and Dawes 1994: 51)

Some of these young people also use alcohol and other drugs to positively assert their cultural differences from their non-indigenous counterparts. In Australia and New Zealand, there have been reports of indigenous young people adopting symbols from the Rastafarian movement, such as reggae music, clothing and dance, along with heavy cannabis use (Davey and Dawes 1994; Durie 2001: 57).

This raises the issue of the cultural determinants of substance use. As Eckersley (2001) points out, social indicators of disadvantage are culturally mediated and some have attempted to explore the role that indigenous cultures play in the patterns of substance use and in interventions. Cultural norms certainly appear to dictate how the community views substance use. In a study of American Indian young people, for example, researchers found that it was only when drinking was seen to interfere with the proper development of cultural values such as courage, humour, generosity and family honour, that it was seen as pathological (O'Nell and Mitchell 1996).

Cultural alienation is frequently cited as a risk factor for much of the ill health of indigenous young people (Brady 1991; Divakaran-Brown and Minutjukur 1993; Durie 2001). However, empirical evidence for this has proved difficult to establish, and there is little convincing evidence that young people who maintain relatively strong links to culture and land are less likely to have problem alcohol and other drug use (Trimble 1998). Young people inhabit complex social and cultural worlds and have to learn to live competently in all of them.

What the above evidence has shown is that use of alcohol and other drugs by indigenous young people cannot simply be explained as an individual characteristic, or even as purely culturally based. Rather, the use of these substances by young people is socially patterned, and relates to their common colonial histories of dispossession and contemporary economic and social marginalisation which is associated the world over with higher rates of alcohol and other drug use. While most non-indigenous young people will moderate their drug taking as they go onto further education, training or employment, indigenous young people have fewer of these opportunities and their expectations are consequently also much lower. This may exacerbate risky drug use.

Programmes and interventions

Like the general population, most indigenous young people do not see their sexual activities or substance use as problematic, and are unlikely to seek help for these behaviours. Substance use generally attracts more attention than the possible ill effects of sexual activity, because of the sometimes immediate consequences of that use, such as alcohol- or other drug-related accidents and violence.

Alcohol and drug policies in each country have had a significant impact on the range and type of interventions. In Australia and New Zealand, harm reduction approaches which acknowledge that drug use and sexual activity are normal aspects of many young people's lives, have been part of national policies directed at minimising the health and social risks of such activity. This includes, for instance, widespread dissemination of safer sex messages and condom distribution. Culturally appropriate messages about moderate drinking are part of regular health promotion and advertising in both New Zealand and Australia (Durie 2001; Saggers and Gray 1998). However, harm reduction policies do not have universal support and many indigenous programmes in both countries insist on an abstinence approach to alcohol and other drug use (Brady 1992). This view is shared by the majority of indigenous communities working on alcohol and other drugs strategies in Canada and the USA, even though harm reduction policies are gradually being introduced in those countries (Health Canada 2001).

Primary prevention of problem substance use – largely through education campaigns and harm reduction strategies among older teenagers and young adults – is more likely to target the general population of young people. Treatment programmes for this group generally include inpatient and hospital-based services, family-based programmes, peer counselling, therapeutic communities and pharmacotherapy. Most are based on the adult chemical dependency model and are usually grounded in the 12-step tradition of Alcoholics Anonymous. Such programmes support identification of the patient as an 'addict' or 'alcoholic' (Lawson and Lawson 1992). It is unclear how acceptable this approach is for many young people, let alone indigenous young people.

In the USA, for example, Thomason (2000) found there were no empirical, research-based findings on the relative efficacy of various treatments for alcohol problems among Native Americans. In our own review of Australian interventions, we found a similar paucity of rigorous evaluations, and weak results at best for those that had been conducted (Gray *et al.* 2000). Importantly, few interventions address in a holistic fashion the known social and cultural determinants of substance use among young people (Loxley *et al.* 2003; Schulenberg and Ebata 1994).

Public health officials and indigenous people stress the importance of addressing the social disadvantage facing indigenous young people, because of their common histories of colonisation, dispossession and marginalisation from mainstream societies (Comeau and Santin 1995; Saggers and Gray 1998; Durie 2001). In particular, increasing the rates of retention at school and participation in the workforce are seen as central to reducing indigenous poverty, ill health, risky sexual behaviour and substance misuse (Chewning *et al.* 2001; Durie 2001; Gray *et al.* 1996).

Family and culture

Although structural factors are implicated in the high rates of problem substance use among indigenous young people, as highlighted earlier, strong families and communities can often protect some young people against the worst effects of such use (Hill and Hill 1992; Durie 2001). For this reason, many indigenous programmes take a whole-of-family approach to addressing problem substance use. Residential alcohol rehabilitation programmes in Canada and Australia, for example, encourage and sometimes require family members to accompany their dependent relatives (Strempel *et al.* 2004; Saggers and Gray 1998). In New Zealand, the Māori concept of *whanauntgatanga* (extended family relationships), along with *whaka-manawa* (encouragement) and *mauri* (spirit) is considered an essential component of Māori counselling (Durie 2001). Usually it is the family, not just the individual, that needs healing.

It is this healing, rather than simply treatment, that many indigenous people are seeking (Durie 2001: 155) and this requires a more holistic approach which incorporates family and culture. Promoting positive indigenous identity, and utilising family-based cultural values are central to cultural models of healing in Australia, Canada, New Zealand and the USA (Durie 2001; Stubben 1997; Saggers and Gray 1998), although they are less well developed in Australia. For instance, there has been a high degree of involvement by the Navajo in the development and implementation of prevention and treatment programmes within communities on their reservation in the USA. Communities were more satisfied with these programmes than previous externally imposed programmes (Stubben 1997). *Mauri* therapy, healing based on Māori concepts, utilises aspects of traditional culture – songs, dance and physical therapies – and has been used to encourage high school students to learn customary values and practices, and more positive health behaviours (Durie 2001).

In South Australia, in one initiative, young petrol sniffers were removed from their families and placed in traditional homelands in the care of a husband and wife team. The aim of the programme was to engage the young people in traditional activities and cultural re-education. Local indigenous people, including parents of sniffers, claim these programmes were successful because: they were owned and controlled by them; parents were happy to hand over their children to the husband and wife team; and young people learned new skills and some did not return to sniffing (Divakaran-Brown and Minutjukur 1993). Again very little is known of the efficacy of these approaches, but they do have wide community support.

There is some evidence that strong integration in both indigenous and Western culture protects against problem substance use (in Stubben 1997). The complex identities held by many indigenous young people mean that health professionals and indigenous communities may need to carefully assess the most appropriate intervention for any individual (Thomason 2000). The attraction that Western culture has for many indigenous young people is a source of conflict in some communities (Brady 1991), but these young people have the right to access all the social and cultural environments available to other citizens.

To address these issues, some bicultural approaches are based on the social and cultural determinants of substance use, and incorporate both Western and indigenous treatment modalities (Young 1992). For instance, the Natitch Salallie Youth Residential Treatment Program in Canada is a combined medical and cultural model of treatment for substance use. It is based on the principle that recovery will occur by building self-esteem through the social, cultural, physical and spiritual holistic approach. Abstinence-based, the programme uses the 12-step approach in individual counselling. Cultural programming is integrated into all aspects of the overall programme and includes compulsory studies into tribal government, tradition and history (NNADAP n.d.).

Conclusions

Having sex and taking drugs are a normal, pleasurable part of growing up in most societies. Young indigenous people engage in these behaviours for the same complex reasons that many people do, but also as part of the process of learning adult behaviour. Attempts to regulate sexual activity and substance use need to differentiate, with indigenous young people themselves, between those behaviours which have few long-term adverse health and social impacts and those which do.

The best protection for indigenous young people is to be part of families and communities which have a strong stake in both their own cultures and communities, and mainstream society. In Australia, Canada, New Zealand and the USA much still needs to be done to symbolically and materially address the injustices of the colonial past, in order to provide indigenous young people with the foundations for health and well being.

Acknowledgements

The National Drug Research Institute, at which Dennis Gray and Phillipa Strempel are employed, is funded by the Australian Government Department of Health and Ageing.

References

Aggleton, P., Ball, A. and Mane, P. (2000) 'Young people, sexuality and relationships', *Sexual and Relationship Therapy* 15: 213–20.

Australia, Department of Health and Family Services (1995) *National drug strategy household survey: Survey report 1995*, Canberra: Australian Government Publishing Service.

Australian Institute of Health and Welfare (AIHW) (2003) *Australia's young people: Their health and wellbeing*, AIHW Cat. No. PHE 50, Canberra: Australian Institute of Health and Welfare.

Beauvais, F. (1992a) 'Trends in Indian adolescent drug and alcohol use', *American Indian and Alaska Native Mental Health Research* 5: 1–12.

Beauvais F. (1992b) 'Comparison of drug use rates for reservation Indian, non-reservation Indian and Anglo youth', *American Indian and Alaska Native Mental Health Research* 5: 13–31.

Beauvais, F. (1992c) 'Drug use of friends: A comparison of reservation and non-reservation Indian youth', *American Indian and Alaska Native Mental Health Research* 5: 43–50.

Beauvais, F., Wayman, J.C., Jumper-Thurman, P., Plested, B. and Helm, H. (2002) 'Inhalant abuse among American Indian and non-Latino white adolescents', *American Journal of Drug and Alcohol Abuse* 28: 171–87.

Blum, R.W., Harmon, B., Harris, L., Bergeisen, L. and Resnick, M.D. (1992) 'American Indian – Alaska Native youth health', *Journal of the American Medical Association* 267: 1637–44.

Brady, M. (1991) *The Health of Young Aborigines*, Hobart: National Clearinghouse for Youth Studies.

Brady, M. (1992) *Heavy metal: The social meaning of petrol sniffing in Australia*, Canberra: Aboriginal Studies Press.

Brady, M. (2002) 'Aborigines and alcohol', *Meanjin* 61: 147–53.

BRC Marketing and Social Research (2003) *Youth and alcohol: 2003 ALAC youth drinking monitor*, Wellington: BRC Marketing and Social Research.

Burbank, V. (1988) *Aboriginal adolescence: Maidenhood in an Australian community*, New Brunswick: Rutgers University Press.

Burger, J. (1987) *Report from the frontier: The state of the world's Indigenous peoples*, London: Zed Books.

Burns, C. and Currie, B.J. (1995) 'Patterns of petrol sniffing and other drug use in young men from an Australian Aboriginal community in Arnhem Land, Northern Territory', *Drug and Alcohol Review* 14: 159–69.

Cashmore, J. (2001) 'Family, early development and the life course: Common risk and protective factors in pathways to prevention', in R. Eckersley, J. Dixon and B. Douglas (eds) *The social origins of health and well-being*, Cambridge: Cambridge University Press.

Cherry, A. (2002) 'Burma (Union of Myanmar)', in A. Cherry, M.E. Dillon and D. Rugh (eds) *Substance abuse: A global view*, Westport, CT: Greenwood Press.

Chewning, B., Douglas, J., Kokotailo, P.K., LaCourt, J., St. Clair, D. and Wilson, D. (2001) 'Protective factors associated with American Indian adolescents' safer sexual patterns', *Maternal and Child Health Journal* 5: 273–80.

Coleman, H., Grant, C. and Collins, J. (2001) 'Inhalant use by Canadian Aboriginal youth', *Journal of Child and Adolescent Substance Abuse* 10: 1–20.

Comeau, P. and Santin, A. (1995) *The first Canadians: A profile of Canada's Native people today*, Toronto: James Lorimer & Company.

Daniels, N., Kennedy, B.P. and Kawachi, I. (1999) 'Why justice is good for our health: The social determinants of health inequalities', *Daedalus* 128: 215–51.

Davey, J. and Dawes, G. (1994) 'What is deviant? A comparison of marijuana usage within Aboriginal and Torres Strait Islander and white Australian youth subcultures', *Youth Studies Australia*, Autumn: 49–52.

Day, P., Sullivan, E.A. and Lancaster, P. (1999) *Indigenous mothers and their babies:*

Australia 1994–1996, AIHW Cat. No. PER-9, Canberra: Australian Institute of Health and Welfare.

Divakaran-Brown, C. and Minutjukur, A. (1993) *Children of dispossession: An evaluation of petrol sniffing on Anangu Pitjantjatjara lands*, Adelaide: The Flinders University of South Australia.

Dunne, M.P., Yeo, M.A. and Keane, J. (2000) 'Substance use by Indigenous and non-Indigenous primary school students', *Australian and New Zealand Journal of Public Health* 24: 546–9.

Durie, M. (1998) *Whaiora: Māori health development*, second edition, Auckland: Oxford University Press.

Durie, M. (2001) *Mauri Ora: The dynamics of Māori health*, Auckland: Oxford University Press.

Eckersley, R. (2001) 'Culture, health and well-being', in R. Eckersley, J. Dixon and B. Douglas (eds) *The social origins of health and well-being*, Cambridge: Cambridge University Press.

Fenwicke, R. and Purdie, G. (2000) 'The sexual activity of 654 fourth form Hawkes Bay students', *New Zealand Medical Journal* 113: 460–4.

Figueroa, L., Infante, P. and Senna P. (2000) *In between the lines: How the New York Times frames youth*, New York: New York City Youth Media Watch.

Forero, R., Bauman, A., Chen, J.X.C. and Flaherty, B. (1999) 'Substance use and socio-demographic factors among Aboriginal and Torres Strait Islander school students in New South Wales', *Australian and New Zealand Journal of Public Health* 23: 295–300.

Gray, D., Morfitt, B., Williams, S., Ryan, K. and Coyne, L. (1996) *Drug use and related issues among young Aboriginal people in Albany*, Perth: National Centre for Research into the Prevention of Drug Abuse, Curtin University of Technology.

Gray, D., Morfitt, B., Williams, S. and Ryan, K. (1997) 'The use of tobacco, alcohol and other drugs by young Aboriginal people in Albany, Western Australia', *Australian and New Zealand Journal of Public Health* 21: 71–6.

Gray, D., Saggers, S., Sputore, B. and Bourbon, D. (2000) 'What works? A review of evaluated alcohol misuse interventions among Aboriginal Australians', *Addiction* 95: 31–42.

Gray, D. and Saggers, S. (2002) 'Indigenous health: the perpetuation of inequality', in J. Germov (ed.) *Second opinion: An introduction to health sociology*, Melbourne: Oxford University Press.

Gray, D., Saggers, S., Atkinson, D., Carter, M., Loxley, W. and Hayward, D. (2001) *The harm reduction needs of Aboriginal people who inject drugs*, Perth: National Drug Research Institute, Curtin University of Technology.

Health Canada (2001) *Reducing the harm associated with injection drug use in Canada*, prepared by F/P/T Advisory Committee on Population Health, F/P/T Committee on Alcohol and Other Drug Issues, F/P/T Advisory Committee on AIDS and F/P/T Heads of Corrections Working Group on HIV/AIDS. For the meeting of Ministers of Health, St John's, Newfoundland, September 2001.

Hill, A. and Hill, V. (1992) 'Substance abuse prevention programs for American Indian youth', in G. Lawson and A. Lawson (eds) *Adolescent Substance Abuse: Etiology, Treatment and Prevention,* Maryland: Aspen Publishers.

Hunter, E. (1993) *Aboriginal health and history*, Melbourne: Cambridge University Press.

Indian Health Service (IHS) (2003) *Trends in Indian Health: 1998–99*, Washington, DC: Indian Health Service.

Johnson, A., Wadsworth, J., Wellings, K. and Field, J. (1994) *Sexual attitudes and lifestyles*, Oxford: Blackwell.

Kawachi, I. (2000) 'Why social epidemiology?' *Australasian Epidemiologist* 7: 5–6.

Kawachi, I., Kennedy, B.P. and Glass, R. (1999) 'Social capital and self-rated health: A contextual analysis', *American Journal of Public Health* 89: 1187–92.

Keating, D.P. and Hertzman, C. (1999) 'Modernity's paradox', in D.P. Keating and C. Hertzman (eds) *Developmental health and the wealth of nations: Social, biological and educational dynamics*, New York: Guilford Press, pp. 1–17.

Kingsbury, K. (1995) '"Indigenous peoples" as an international concept', in R.H. Barnes, A. Gray and B. Kingsbury (eds) *Indigenous peoples of Asia*, Ann Arbor, Michigan: The Association for Asian Studies, pp. 13–34.

Larsen, S. and Saglie, J. (1996) 'Alcohol use in Saami and non-Saami areas in northern Norway', *European Addiction Research* 3: 78–82.

Larson, A., Shannon, C., Brough, M. and Eldridge, C. (1997) *Indigenous youth, alcohol and other drugs,* IDU working paper 3, Brisbane: University of Queensland, Australian Centre for International and Tropical Health and Nutrition.

Larson, A., Shannon, C. and Eldridge, C. (1999) 'Indigenous Australians who inject drugs: Results from a Brisbane study', *Drug and Alcohol Review* 18: 53–62.

Lawson, G. and Lawson, A. (eds) (1992) *Adolescent substance abuse: Etiology, treatment and prevention*, Gaithersburg, MD: Aspen Publishers.

Loxley, W., Toumbourou, J.W., Stockwell, T., Haines, B., Scott, K., Godfrey, C., Waters, E., Patton, G., Forham, R., Gray, D., Marshall, J., Ryder, D., Saggers, S., Sanci, L. and Williams, J. (2003) *The prevention of substance use, risk and harm in Australia: A review of the evidence*, Canberra: Ministerial Council on Drug Strategy.

Lynch, J. (2000) 'Social epidemiology: Some observations from the past, present and future', *Australasian Epidemiologist* 7: 7–15.

Lynskey, M. and Fergusson, D. (1993) 'Sexual activity and contraceptive use amongst teenagers under the age of 15 years', *New Zealand Medical Journal* 106: 511–14.

Marmot, M. and Wilkinson, R.G. (1999) *Social determinants of health*, Oxford: Oxford University Press.

May, P.A. and Moran, J.R. (1995) 'Prevention of alcohol misuse: a review of health promotion efforts among American Indians', *Journal of Primary Prevention* 22: 201–33.

Morris, L., Warren, C.W. and Aral, S.O. (1993) 'Measuring adolescent sexual behaviours and related health outcomes', *Public Health Reports* 108: 31–5.

Najman, J. (2001) 'A general model of the social origins of health and well-being', in R. Eckersley, J. Dixon and B. Douglas (eds) *The social origins of health and well-being*, Cambridge: Cambridge University Press.

National Native Alcohol and Drug Abuse Program (NNADAP) (n.d.) *Evaluation strategies in Aboriginal substance abuse programs: A discussion*, Ontario: Health Canada. Online. Available HTTP: <www.hc-sc.gc.ca/fnihb-dgspni/fnihb/cp/nnadap/publications/>

New Zealand, Ministry of Health, Manatu Hauroa (1995) *Cannabis: Public Health Issues 1995–1996*, Wellington: Ministry of Health.

Oetting, E.R., Beauvais, F. and Edwards, R. (1988) 'Alcohol and Indian youth: Social and psychological correlates and prevention', *Journal of Drug Issues* 18: 87–101.

O'Nell, T.D. and Mitchell, C.M. (1996) 'Alcohol use among American Indian adolescents: The role of culture in pathological drinking', *Social Science and Medicine* 42: 565–78.

Pearson, G. (1983) *Hooligan: A history of respectable fears*, London: Macmillan.

Pool, I., Dickson, J., Dharmalingham, A., Hillcoat-Nalletamby, S., Johnstone, K. and Roberts, H. (1999) *New Zealand's contraceptive revolutions,* ISM, Population Studies Centre, University of Waikato.

Rice, F.P. (1996) *The adolescent: Development, relationships, and culture*, eighth edition, Boston: Allyn & Bacon.

Saggers, S. and Gray, D. (1991) *Aboriginal health and society*, Sydney: Allen & Unwin.

Saggers, S. and Gray, D. (1998) *Dealing with alcohol: Indigenous usage in Australia, New Zealand and Canada*, Melbourne: Cambridge University Press.

Schulenberg, J. and Ebata, A.T. (1994) 'The United States', in K. Hurrelmann (ed.) *International Handbook of Adolescence*, Westport: Greenwood Press.

Schultes, R.E. (1990) 'An overview of hallucinogens in the Western hemisphere', in P.T. Furst (ed.) *Flesh of the gods: The ritual use of hallucinogens*, second edition, Prospect Heights, IL: Waveland Press Inc.

Sercombe, H. (1997) *Naming youth: The construction of the youth category*, Unpublished PhD thesis, Perth: Murdoch University.

Shoobridge, J. (1998) 'The health and psychological consequences of injecting drug use in an Aboriginal community', in K. Dyer and D. Addy (eds) *New perspectives: Proceedings of the 1997 NCETA Research Seminar Program*, Bedford Park, SA: National Centre for Education and Training in Addiction.

Social Exclusion Unit (1999) *Teenage pregnancy – Report to Parliament*, United Kingdom.

Spooner, C., Hall, W. and Lynskey, M. (2001) *Structural determinants of youth drug use*, Woden, ACT: Australian National Council on Drugs.

Statistics New Zealand, Te Tari Tatau (1998) *New Zealand now: Young New Zealanders*, Wellington: Statistics New Zealand.

Strempel, P., Saggers, S., Gray, D. and Stearne, A. (2004) *Indigenous drug and alcohol projects: Elements of best practice*, Canberra: Australian National Council on Drugs.

Stubben, J. (1997) 'Culturally competent substance abuse prevention research among rural Native American communities', in E.B. Robertson, Z. Sloboda, G.M. Boyd, L. Beatty and N.J. Kozel (eds) *Rural substance abuse: State of knowledge and issues*, NIDA Research Monograph 168, Rockville, MD: National Institute on Drug Abuse.

Symonds, P. (1998) 'Political economy and cultural logics of HIV/AIDS among the Hmong of Northern Thailand', in M. Singer (ed.) *The political economy of AIDS*, Amityvill, NY: Baywood.

Thomason, T. (2000) 'Issues in the treatment of Native Americans with alcohol problems', *Journal of Multicultural Counselling and Development*, 28: 243–52.

Trewin, D. and Madden, R. (2003) *The health and welfare of Australia's Aboriginal and Torres Strait Islander peoples: 2003*, Canberra: Australian Bureau of Statistics.

Trimble, J.E. (1998) 'Cultural diversity and influences on drinking behaviour', *Journal of the Alcoholic Beverage Medical Research Foundation* 8. 45–9.

United Nations Commission on Human Rights, Sub-Commission on Prevention of Discrimination and Protection of Minorities (1994) 'Draft Declaration on the Rights of Indigenous Peoples', in van der Vlist, L. (ed.) *Voices of the earth*, Amsterdam: International Books/NCIP, Appendix II, pp. 305–16.

Young, R.S. (1992) *Review of treatment strategies for Native American alcoholics: The need for a cultural perspective*, Tucson, AZ: University of Arizona.

Index